# PERSON-CENTERED COMMUNICATION WITH OLDER ADULTS

# PERSON-CENTERED COMMUNICATION WITH OLDER ADULTS
## The Professional Provider's Guide

TIMOTHY A. STORLIE, PhD

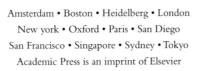

Amsterdam • Boston • Heidelberg • London
New york • Oxford • Paris • San Diego
San Francisco • Singapore • Sydney • Tokyo
Academic Press is an imprint of Elsevier

Academic Press is an imprint of Elsevier
125 London Wall, London EC2Y 5AS, UK
525 B Street, Suite 1800, San Diego, CA 92101-4495, USA
225 Wyman Street, Waltham, MA 02451, USA
The Boulevard, Langford Lane, Kidlington, Oxford OX5 1GB, UK

**Notices**
Knowledge and best practice in this field are constantly changing. As new research and
experience broaden our understanding, changes in research methods, professional practices,
or medical treatment may become necessary.

Practitioners and researchers must always rely on their own experience and knowledge in
evaluating and using any information, methods, compounds, or experiments described
herein. In using such information or methods they should be mindful of their own safety
and the safety of others, including parties for whom they have a professional responsibility.

To the fullest extent of the law, neither the Publisher nor the authors, contributors, or
editors, assume any liability for any injury and/or damage to persons or property as a
matter of products liability, negligence or otherwise, or from any use or operation of any
methods, products, instructions, or ideas contained in the material herein.

ISBN: 978-0-12-420132-3

**British Library Cataloguing in Publication Data**
A catalogue record for this book is available from the British Library

**Library of Congress Catalog Number**
A catalog record for this book is available from the Library of Congress

For information on all Academic Press publications
visit our website at http://store.elsevier.com/

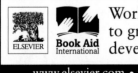

Working together
to grow libraries in
developing countries

www.elsevier.com • www.bookaid.org

Typeset by TNQ Books and Journals
www.tnq.co.in

Printed and bound in the United States of America

# DEDICATION

For the prolific author Frances J. Storlie, my mom and professional role-model. For my dad Alton H. Storlie, who spent endless summer afternoons with me engaged in intergenerational-communication.

For my wife Debra Belshee-Storlie—an extraordinary woman and gifted psychologist—whose unwavering belief in me, content contributions, and editorial assistance played a huge role in bringing this manuscript to completion. For my son Martin R. Storlie—a bright and intensely driven young business man—whose personal example of self-discipline helped provide me with the motivation needed to finish this book.

For my good friends and authors, George D. Zgourides and Loren W. Christensen who encouraged me and provided many valuable tips about the publication process.

For world-class scholars and mentors, the late Dr. Jeanne Achterberg, Dr. Stanley Krippner, and Dr. Steven Pritzker whose collective body of work is truly inspirational and who were instrumental in the development of my research and writing skills. For Dr. Jon Nussbaum for taking the time to read my manuscript and write the Foreword.

For Emily, Barbara, and Edward—three outstanding professionals from Elsevier who supported the concept for this book and helped bring it to publication.

And for all elders—especially my grandfather.

# CONTENTS

## 6. Person-Centered Communication: Age-Related Changes, Cultural Challenges, and Difficult Conversations     87

**Core Question:** How can the person-centered communication approach assist the provider when discussing sensitive issues with older adults, when interacting with older adults from another culture, and/or when interacting with older adults suffering from hearing loss, aphasia, or dementia?     87

    The Eighth C—Calmness**                                      **109**

    **Core Question:** How can the person-centered communication approach help
       lower frustration and stress for both the provider and older adult?    109

    Introduction: The Stress of Communication                         109
    Poor Communication and Stress                                     110
    The Body's Stress Response                                        111
    The Experience of Stress: Fight-or-Flight or Tend-and-Befriend    111
    Definitions of Stress                                             112
    The Stress Response                                               113
    Resilience                                                       113
    Do No Harm Revisited                                             114
    Provider Stress                                                  114
    Community Living, Stress, and the Older Adult                     114
    Stressors                                                        115
    Common Occupational Stressors                                    115
    Professional Burnout                                             116
    Effects of Staff Burnout on Quality of Services                  117
    Stress and the Provider's Personal Plan of Care                  118
    The Key Role of Organization Administration                      118
    Stress Plan of Care for the Provider                             120
    Defusing Stress: Eliciting the Relaxation Response               120
    Time Out for the Professional                                    123
    The Stress of Commuting                                          124
    The Stress of Documentation                                      124
    Conclusion                                                       125
    List of Main Points for Preview and Review                       126
    Web Resources                                                    128
    References                                                       128

8.  **Person-Centered Communication: Mental Imagery and
    Imagined Interactions**                                           **131**

    **Core Question:** How can mental imagery be used to improve the quality of
       provider/older adult interpersonal communication?             131

    Introduction                                                     131
    Evidence for the Efficacy of Imagery                             132
    Learning Curves and Developmental Trajectories                   132
    Historical Use of Mental Imagery                                 132

# FOREWORD

Dr. Storlie has authored a book solidly grounded within the person-centered approach toward communication. He offers pragmatic suggestions that will help improve the communication competencies for professionals serving older adults. The book eloquently provides guidance that will improve the quality of the communication between healthcare professionals and their older adult clients. Providing health care to older adults involves a multidisciplinary approach. Each professional across numerous professional disciplines can improve her or his communicative competence by following the suggestions provided within this book. In addition, the communicative changes recommended will not only improve the quality of care provided to older adults but will also lead to a much higher level of satisfaction in providing that care and to a higher quality of life for their older adult clients.

Healthcare providers are often younger than the older adults they serve. One of the enduring myths held by many is that we, as providers, can competently interact with all of our patients/clients. The majority of us feel that intergenerational interactions are no more challenging than interactions within our own age group. After all, we think, I can communicate easily with my grandparents, parents, children, and grandchildren and am very satisfied within those relationships.

To the surprise of most individuals, even to those well educated within the social sciences, our research has consistently shown that intergenerational communication is very difficult. Miscommunication within the healthcare provider and older adult patient interaction is a frequent and significant contributor to bad health outcomes. This miscommunication is not only caused by ageism but often intensifies the problem of ageism within our society. Healthcare clinics and institutions are some of the worst environments (by this I mean the most ageist) where intergenerational communication between relatively young healthcare workers and older adults is rampant, and it presents a serious impediment to competent delivery of quality health services.

I am often asked why I have spent my entire scholarly/academic career investigating the lives of older adults. Forty years ago, my chosen area of concentration (developmental psychology) rarely produced scholars who focused on anything outside of the first 12 years of life. As a matter of fact, the best theories of human development were certain that all significant positive accomplishments within the brain, or of various socialization processes (learn-ing, parenting, etc.) outside the brain, occur many years before our twentieth birthday. If the various critical periods for brain development or social/moral development were not achieved early in life, then these critical human accom-plishments were determined not to emerge. Old age was a time of depriva-tion and loss, not worthy of scholarly investigation or healthcare energy.

The universal demographic shift toward an older population with longer lifespans, the discovery of brain plasticity, and the realization that individuals can continue to achieve positive developmental changes across both physical and psychosocial domains throughout their entire lifespans have created a new interest in older adulthood, focused upon a more complete under-standing of the aging process. In addition, we have realized that competent social interactions and relationships within both family/friendships and within formal/professional settings constructed through our communica-tion were as important to our overall quality of life throughout the entire lifespan as our biological or physiological well-being.

As individuals develop throughout their lifespan, significant changes do occur within the domains of biology, physiology, psychology, sociology, spiri-tuality, and technology. These changes can often lead to a slow deterioration in our cognitive and communicative abilities. At the same time, our experiences, changes/modifications in the physical structure of our built environment, a growing or a maintaining of the social network of close family and friends, and advances in technology help us to achieve a high quality of life well into our eighth decade. Perhaps, the most important two realizations—that our brain has plasticity (can learn and change as we age) and that our brain is so big because it has evolved to ensure that we are social beings—have provided a solid foundation to be a tad more optimistic about the aging process. We age *with* others and are not meant to age in isolation.

Older adulthood is an important and significant time in the life of an individual, and providers are in the unique position of being able to help improve the quality of life for older adults by providing superior services. This book identifies the provider–older adult relationship and communica-tion as the very core of providing excellent care.

Jon F. Nussbaum Ph.D.
Professor of Communication Arts & Sciences
and Human Development and Family Studies
The Pennsylvania State University

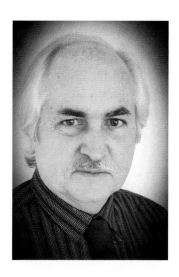

# ABOUT THE AUTHOR

Timothy A. Storlie, MS, MSW, PhD, is a psychologist, licensed counselor, and medical social worker. With nearly 20 years of gerontological-oriented professional experience, Dr Storlie has provided person-centered counseling to hundreds of older adults. He developed a county-wide program to instruct older adults on how to use public transportation, served on an interdisciplinary team charged with investigating cases of suspected elder abuse, and conducted assessments of older adults residing in skilled care nursing facilities.

As a medical social worker, Dr Storlie provided communication-related training for the staff of several home health and hospice agencies, facilitated bereavement support groups, consulted with physicians and nurses on how to improve provider–patient relations, and developed a reminiscence-based program for use by hospice patients entitled *Defining Moments*. Dr Storlie was a popular community college adjunct instructor where for 10 years he taught a "standing-room-only" course entitled *Therapeutic Communication for the Health Professional*. In addition to writing, counseling, and teaching, he enjoys coaching doctoral students majoring in counseling, gerontology, psychology, or social work.

Committed to reducing ageism, Dr Storlie is a passionate advocate for the person-centered approach to communication between providers and older adults. He serves as an expert member and field editor of the Social

Trends section of TechCast Global—a research organization that produces authoritative forecasts designed to help governments, businesses and organizations adapt to a rapidly changing world. A Fellow of the American Stress Institute, his current research interests include stress and health in older adults, mind-body-medicine and longevity in the older patient, integrative medical and mental health care, online counseling, and establishing jargon-free, plain language standards for human services professionals.

Dr Storlie graduated from Saybrook University where he earned a PhD in Psychology with a dual concentration—Integrative Health Studies and Consciousness and Spirituality. His dissertation was nominated for the Dissertation of Distinction Award. He also completed a postdoctoral certificate in Dream Studies. Prior to receiving his doctorate, he completed a BS in Education from Portland State University and two graduate degrees also from PSU—an MS in Special Education and an MSW in Social Work. Dr Storlie is a nationally certified, WA State Licensed Mental Health Counselor, Registered Hypnotherapist, and Certified Master Level Trainer in NLP. www.Person-CenteredCommunicationwithOlderAdults.Com.

# PREFACE

Providers serving adults of age 65 and above face a growing problem—older adults are becoming increasingly dissatisfied with the quality of services. The two reasons most often cited for this dissatisfaction are poor quality communication and unsatisfactory provider relationships. This book was written to address this problem. Directed both to the providers of today and for the educators who help prepare the providers of tomorrow, it recommends providers adopt an evidence-based, collaborative, empathic, plain-language, person-centered approach to communication. To further enhance the quality of communication, the author recommends providers adhere to 10 overarching principles referred to as the 10 "C's"—caring, compassionate, courteous, clear, concise, congruent, complete, calm, coherent, and connected. Improved communication encourages mutual respect and understanding, enhances the accurate exchange of information, positively impacts outcomes of interactions, increases compliance with provider recommendations, improves older adult satisfaction with service delivery, and decreases older adult complaints and lawsuits. It can also enhance employee retention, lower organizational costs associated with staff turnover, and help reduce the frustration and stress often experienced by both the provider and older adult.

Those working with older adults have an ethical responsibility to "do no harm." Providers who adopt a plain-language approach reduce the risk of inflicting unintentional harm. Misunderstandings can lead to unpleasant consequences. As 70% of medical litigations are related to unsatisfactory communication between doctors and patients, this can be an important benefit.

The topic of communication is deep and wide. The skills required for accurate, effective, and mutually satisfying communication are many. A prime objective of this book is to invite providers to cultivate a perspective of aging and older adults that fosters a more respectful, person-centered style of communication. To assist with this endeavor, Chapter 2 is devoted to the topic of "how to learn." It presents a systematic learning strategy for approaching the information, knowledge, and practices contained in the rest of the book. Employing these strategies, planning suggestions, goal-setting techniques, and implementation methods should prove helpful to providers developing a person-centered approach to communicating.

Rare to this genre, this book introduces providers to three underappreciated and underdiscussed topics within the field of communication. First, the role of mental imagery in the communication process is described and providers are shown how imagery can be used to help develop person-centered communication skills and lower stress. Second, providers are introduced to exciting new research findings from the field of neurocardiology. These findings describe how the brain and heart mutually influence each other and interact during the communication process. They suggest that the heart's cardioelectromagnetic field may be a source of information exchange between individuals. Providers are shown how the experience of positive emotions, such as appreciation or compassion, may enhance cortical functioning and communication ability. Finally, controversial findings from research in three concepts from quantum physics—*entanglement, nonlocality,* and *distance intentionality*—are presented. Methods for applying these concepts to potentially enhance the quality of interpersonal communication are explored.

Approximately 100 billion people have lived on earth. The current population of over 7 billion, includes 531 million individuals of age 65 or older—the fastest growing population segment. Numerous services for older adults are provided by a vast array of agencies, organizations, facilities, and programs, collectively referred to as the aging services network. Service is rendered via millions of providers, such as directors, program and case managers, doctors, nurses, and a multitude of staff and volunteers—all dedicated to addressing the needs, concerns, and problems of older adults.

Unfortunately, there exists an increasing dissatisfaction with the quality of service delivery among older adults. Factors contributing to this problem include the following:

1. Many providers need improvement with communication skills.
2. Many providers are not fully aware of the benefits of adopting a person-centered approach to service delivery.
3. Many providers continue to use overly complex, professional jargon.
4. Many providers hold ageist attitudes or use ageist language.
5. Many providers fail to respect cultural differences and also fail to recognize age-related changes that can impede the communication process.

There are many barriers to effective, person-centered communication. One of the biggest barriers is ageism—the tendency to negatively stereotype older adults, display prejudice, and discriminate against individuals simply because they are older. Ageism is a dehumanizing and demoralizing cross-cultural social problem that affects millions of individuals. It is especially prevalent in the United States. In its worst form, ageism leads to physical, emotional, mental, or financial abuse. Other potential communication challenges discussed in this book include lack of knowledge or misunderstandings about age-related changes, cultural differences, stress, and the difficulties of addressing emotionally laden, sensitive topics.

One of the more useful features of this book are the opening "core questions" posed at the beginning of each of the 11 chapters. This core question encourages purposeful reading and provides a solid conceptual foundation upon which new learning and skills may take shape. The 11 core questions include the following:

- Why do so many older adults feel dissatisfied with the quality of their provider relationships and how can providers reduce this dissatisfaction?
- How can providers learn and implement the person-centered approach to interpersonal communication?
- How can a provider develop a respectful, person-centered relationship with an older adult?
- What are the main characteristics of effective, respectful, person-centered communication?
- What is ageism and how does it impact the older adult, the provider–older adult relationship, and the person-centered approach to communication?
- How can the person-centered communication approach assist the provider when discussing sensitive issues with older adults, when interacting with older adults from another culture, and/or when interacting with older adults suffering from hearing loss, aphasia, or dementia?
- How can the person-centered communication approach help lower frustration and stress for both the provider and older adult?
- How can mental imagery be used to improve the quality of provider/ older adult interpersonal communication?
- How can a provider use findings from the field of neurocardiology to enhance the person-centered, interpersonal communication process?
- How can a provider use information from the field of quantum physics to enhance the person-centered, interpersonal communication process?
- How might a person-centered, interpersonal communication approach benefit the providers and older adults of the hi-tech future?

Additional learning aids include practical examples, case studies, provider exercises, a summary of each chapter's main points that can be used both for previewing and reviewing, and a list of resources and references for further learning. Each chapter includes a provider self-test that can also serve as a list of discussion suggestions for instructors.

The elders of the future, similar to their counterparts today, will almost certainly prefer service-oriented relationships with empathic providers who treat them with respect—professionals committed to a person-centered approach to communication. The hope is that—as the Internet of People and the Internet of Things continues to intertwine, and the partnership of head and heart continues to deepen and mature—humanity will feel more connected and compassionate with the population of older adults and, as a result, become more human, not less.

Timothy A. Storlie

# CHAPTER 1

# Providers, Older Adults, and Communication

*I ka olelo ke ola, ika olelo ka make.*
*In the word there is life; in the word there is death.*

**Ancient Hawaiian Saying (Charcot, 1983)**

**Core Question:** Why do so many older adults feel dissatisfied with the quality of their provider relationships, and how can providers reduce this dissatisfaction?

**Keywords:** Ageism; Baby boomer; Communication; Older adult; Person-centered; Plain language; Professional jargon; Respect.

## INTRODUCTION

Words are potent. Within the sprawling aging services network, millions of providers interact with millions of older adults on a regular basis. During these professional interactions, each enters into a dance of words and gestures—a dance that conveys information (Dossey, 2011). This dance transmits meaning—meaning that can encourage or discourage, reassure or frighten. The purpose of this book is to encourage providers to use words purposefully—mindful of their power to help or harm the older adult.

Older adults (individuals age 65 or older) are the fastest growing segment of the population in the United States and globally (U.S. Bureau of the Census, 2011). This increase—due in part to the generation of baby boomers born between 1946 and 1964—is expected to continue until 2030 and significantly impact most aspects of society and the related network of service providers.

Growing numbers of older adults are voicing dissatisfaction with service providers (Greene & Burleson, 2003). The main reasons cited are the poor quality of the provider/older adult relationships and unsatisfactory interpersonal communication. Unsatisfactory communication can impact the quality of services rendered as well as service outcomes.

*Person-Centered Communication with Older Adults*
http://dx.doi.org/10.1016/B978-0-12-420132-3.00001-5

1

Ineffective, unsatisfactory communication has many causes. This chapter introduces five major causes that will be the focus of much discussion throughout this book:

1. Underdeveloped provider communication skills.
2. Lack of provider commitment to a person-centered service delivery approach.
3. Inappropriate use of professional jargon by providers.
4. Ageist attitudes and language by the provider.
5. Impediments to effective communication stemming from cultural differences and from age-related physical, social, and psychological changes in the older adult.

This book argues for a person-centered, respect-based, Plain Language approach to communicating with older adults. It explains how providers can communicate more effectively, more respectfully, and less stressfully.

Providing services to older adults can be rewarding, yet stressful (Tamparo & Lindh, 2008). Communication between providers and older adults is often perceived as demanding and challenging (Hart, 2010). Improved communication can deepen rapport, increase mutual respect and understanding, enhance accurate exchange of information, improve compliance with provider recommendations, positively impact outcomes, and often save time while lowering frustration and stress for the provider and the older adult.

## A MESSAGE TO SERVICE PROVIDERS

Do older adults (individuals aged 65 or older) comprise a significant percentage of your patient, client, or customer base? Is communicating with older adults a regular and frequent part of your work? Are older adults one of the target groups for your practice, agency, or program?

Are you an educator helping students to prepare for a career that includes working with older adults? If you answered "yes" to any of the preceding questions, this book was written for you.

## EVERY OLDER ADULT HAS A HISTORY AND A STORY—HERE IS FRANCES'S

The medication aide at the assisted living facility—a thirty-something woman with two years of professional experience—glared at Frances and impatiently demanded she sit down and take her to prescribed medications. Eighty-eight-year-old Frances, a relatively new resident at the facility, complied and choked back her tears just long enough to return to the privacy of her apartment where she sat and cried off and on for the next hour.

As a pioneering nurse practitioner with a Ph.D., Frances had served thousands of patients during her long medical career. She helped establish intensive care units around the United States, taught in university nursing programs, served as keynote speaker for several national professional association meetings, and was the recipient of various prestigious professional awards.

A published poet and author of seven nursing-related text books and 112 professional journal articles, Frances completed over 45 medical mission trips to Central and South America since she retired. Today, she was being ordered where to sit and told what to do by a near-total stranger who was young enough to be her granddaughter—a stranger who knew next to nothing of her lifetime of professional achievements.

Frances finished describing her many accomplishments. She wiped away her tears, looked directly into my eyes and said, "Tim, I'd trade it all—all of it—for some old-fashioned human kindness, a little courtesy and respect" (personal conversation, 2013).

Unfortunately, Frances's experience is not atypical. Her example showcases a major problem in the United States—the problem of disrespect often shown to older adults in a service-delivery system that is more frequently provider centered than person centered. During my experience as a home health and hospice medical social worker, I observed dozens of similar cases and situations where a patient, client, or resident was treated disrespectfully, interactions where each individual wanted only what Frances had wanted—a precious minute or two of another's attention, given with kindness and respect.

## THE OLDER ADULT WANTS WHAT EVERY PERSON WANTS

Ideally—in an atmosphere of person-centered services—the older adult's interests and needs remain central. Whether the older adults served by providers are called patients, clients, residents, customers, or consumers, they are—underneath all labels—unique individuals, each with a special story, a specific past, current conditions, and future aspirations.

The provider's task is simple (yet frequently challenging): Keep the needs of the older adult as the central focus of service and see, hear, and interact with the individual as a unique person and not as a "patient," "client," or "customer." Drench, Noonan, Sharby, and Ventura (2012) suggest that before taking action, the provider ask, "What are the client's needs and how will this help him or her?" (p. 5).

In every encounter, older adults want to be seen for who they are, listened to and heard, respected and appreciated. Each wants to feel as if she or he matters enough for the provider to offer a few minutes of undivided attention.

## OLDER ADULTS—THE FASTEST GROWING SEGMENT OF THE GLOBAL POPULATION

From the birth of the first human being until today (2014), approximately 100 billion people have lived on earth. Over seven billion are presently alive. Of these, 531 million individuals are estimated to be aged 65 or older (U.S. Bureau of the Census, 2010). Projections indicate this number could double by 2030 and reach 1.53 billion by 2050.

On January 1, 2011, the first of the baby boom generation (individuals born between 1946 and 1964) turned aged 65. Every day since then, another 10,000 American baby boomers have celebrated their 65th birthday— approximately one every 8.6 s (http://www.pewsocialtrends.org). These numbers emphasize the magnitude of the impact that these changing demographics will likely have on society and the network of aging service providers.

## STRAIN ON HEALTHCARE, SOCIAL SERVICES PROGRAMS, AND PROVIDERS

The unprecedented increase in the population of older adults will continue unabated until 2030. At that point, approximately one out of every five Americans will be 65 or older (U.S. Department of Health and Human Services, 2013).

The sheer numbers of "boomers" reaching their 65th birthday will likely exert significant strains on the healthcare and other social services systems, impact millions of individual providers, and influence most aspects of American society.

## THE EXPANDING NETWORK OF PROVIDERS OF SERVICES TO OLDER ADULTS

Globally, there are over 59 million people who work in healthcare (World Healthcare Organization, 2014). In the United States, the healthcare sector—where more than 18 million individuals are employed—is one of the fastest growing areas of the US economy (Centers for Disease Control and Prevention, 2014).

To address the needs of an expanding population base of older adults, the network of service providers—the vast array of agencies, organizations, and professionals that focus all or part of their activities on meeting the needs of older people—is also expanding. This diverse network includes but is not limited to the following:

- Medical doctors, physician's assistants, pharmacists, and nurses.
- Psychiatrists, psychologists, social workers, and counselors.
- Chaplains, ministers, rabbis, and priests.
- Physical, occupational, speech, respiratory, music, and massage therapists.
- Ophthalmologists and optometrists.
- Dentists and dental hygienists.
- Audiologists and hearing aid counselors.
- Various medical and lab technicians, medical assistants, home health aides, medical equipment providers, transportation providers, and food service workers.
- Naturopathic physicians, chiropractors, podiatrists, and acupuncturists.
- Elder law attorneys, ombudsman, and adult protective services investigators.
- Directors, program managers, coordinators, case managers, board members, and volunteers of older adult programs and agencies.
- Directors, supervisors, and staff of skilled care nursing, assisted living, adult day care, recreational, and respite care facilities.
- Professors, instructors, and educators who teach aging-related courses to help prepare future providers of older adult services.

## AUTHOR COMMENT: COMMUNICATION—THE COMMON THREAD

The members of the network of older adult service providers deserve recognition and appreciation. They perform an invaluable service yet are often overworked, underpaid, and underappreciated.

The author—a former hospice medical social worker and licensed mental health counselor—served on several interdisciplinary healthcare teams. This provided rich experience collaborating and consulting with members from most of the preceding named professional categories and—more importantly—hundreds of older adults.

The common thread connecting my colleagues—as well as the providers listed above—is that each of them regularly communicated with older adults. At one time or another, most spoke of the personal satisfaction felt from providing needed services, while also acknowledging the stress that frequently accompanied provider–older adult interactions. Over the years, many interesting questions were raised, such as the following:

- Why do so many older adults feel unhappy with their providers?
- How can providers cultivate effective working relationships with older adults?
- How can providers become more person centered when caring for older adults?
- What are the main characteristics of effective, respectful, person-centered communication?
- What are some of the common barriers to effective communication?
- How can a provider enhance the communication process when interacting with an older adult suffering from age-related hearing loss?
- What impact does aphasia have on an older adult's ability to speak and understand another person's language?
- What are some of the ways a provider can enhance the communication process when speaking with an older adult who has Alzheimer's disease?
- How can providers reduce or eliminate the use of professional jargon when speaking with older adults?
- What impact do ageist language and attitudes have on older adults?
- How can providers reduce personal stress?
- How can mental imagery be used to improve the quality of interpersonal communications with older adults?
- How can recent findings from neurocardiology and physics be used to enhance interpersonal communication?
- What technological advances are predicted for the near future that could improve the quality of life for the twenty-first century older adult?

This book offers practical information and evidence-based suggestions to help address these and many other communication-related questions and challenges. It is not a book on how to do psychotherapy nor is it a book on human development. The focus of this book is how to improve professional-level communication and lower the stress often experienced both by providers and by the patients, clients, and customers they serve.

## THE CORE PROBLEM: DISSATISFACTION WITH PROVIDER COMMUNICATION

Effective communication is central to an individual's capacity for functioning as a member of society. A key aspect of all relationships when they break down, and the most frequent complaint, relates to poor communication (Phelps & Hassed, 2012).

Communication is "a process by which information is exchanged between individuals through a common system of symbols, signs, or behavior" (Mish, 2009, p. 251). Studies suggest that the style of communication used between providers and older adults can significantly impact the service quality that the older adult receives and influence resulting outcomes (Greene & Burleson, 2003).

Research into healthcare communication between providers and older adults has progressed rapidly over the past 20 years. Knapp and Daly (2011) point out that the outcome most frequently measured is patient satisfaction. A large percentage of older adults have become increasingly dissatisfied with provider relationships (Greene & Burleson, 2003). Interestingly, the technical incompetence of the professional is rarely cited as the reason for this dissatisfaction. Most often cited is the quality of the provider relationship and the quality of the interpersonal communication—especially how well understood the older adult feels. Phelps and Hassed (2012) report that in the medical arena, unsatisfactory communication between doctors and patients is the leading factor in 70% of related litigations.

## THE HIGH COSTS OF MISCOMMUNICATION AND MISUNDERSTANDING

Small mistakes can take place daily when communicating with older adults. Some are as simple as calling the older adult by the wrong name, others are more complicated (Sheldon, 2004). For example, older adults account for approximately 34% of all prescription drug use in the United States. The U.S. Centers for Disease Control and Prevention report that two-thirds of older adults are unable to comprehend the information provided about their prescription medications (Gerontology News, May 2014).

For the older adult, the "cost" of poor, ineffective communication may be physical, emotional, psychological, monetary, or involve increased stress and health risks. For the provider, the cost may be an increase in stress and frustration, loss of professional credibility, loss of revenue—even the loss of employment or the right to practice.

Miscommunication can lead to misunderstandings and misinterpretations. Misunderstandings can lead to dissatisfaction, hurt feelings, delays in needed services, increased risks, and lost provider revenues. Misunderstandings can cost but mistakes can be even more costly—especially those leading to increased risk to health or litigation. Hospital error is the third largest cause of death in the United States (James, 2013). Providers can reduce the risk of misunderstanding by adopting a person-centered, effective, respectful, Plain-Talk approach to communicating with older adults.

## POOR COMMUNICATION AND STRESS

Problems arising from interpersonal communication can be stressful. Chronically elevated levels of stress can negatively impact the older adult, the provider, and, if applicable, even his or her employer. For the older adult, excessive stress can result in an increased interpersonal conflict, reduced satisfaction with provider services, poorer therapeutic outcomes, and increased health risks.

For the provider, chronic overexposure to stress may lead to interpersonal conflicts, reduced morale, increased absenteeism, increased health risks, and professional burnout. For the employer, the negative impact of stressful communications can lead to problems with staff relations, reduced quality of services, increases in client dissatisfaction, problems with staff retention, and increased expenses related to employee turnover.

## CORE BARRIERS TO EFFECTIVE COMMUNICATION

This chapter identifies five core barriers to effective, mutually satisfying communication between providers and older adults:

1. Underdeveloped professional communication skills: Professional communication skills include cultivating rapport, use of observation and listening, mindfulness, and asking questions to name a few.

2. Lack of commitment to a person-centered service delivery system: A person-centered approach, in contrast to a provider-centered approach, places the needs of the older adult ahead of those of the provider.

3. Inappropriate use of professional jargon: Overly complex, technical terms are often confusing and counterproductive to respectful, person-centered communication.

4. Ageist attitudes and language: Ageism centers around the concept of discrimination based on a person's age. It is based on myths and stereotypes about aging, combined with language that evokes negative impressions of older adults. Ageism has been identified as a pervasive problem in Western societies (Williams & Nussbaum, 2001, p. 55). Ageist attitudes and language can significantly impact the quality of communication and

the quality of the relationship between a provider and older adult. Ageism is to old age what racism is to skin color and sexism is to gender. In its worst form, ageism leads to elder abuse, mistreatment, and neglect (Robnett & Chop, 2010).

5. Challenges stem from cultural differences and age-related physical, social, and psychological changes.

## PROFESSIONAL REFLECTION

Providers are encouraged to spend time reflecting on their professional experience associated with communicating with older adults, contemplating questions such as the following:

- Is your professional experience communicating with older adults mostly person centered, effective, respectful, and mutually satisfying? If so, why? What are you doing and/or not doing that is creating this satisfying experience? List some of the main qualities, characteristics, or skills that contribute to your success. Identify any areas that need improvement.

- If your overall experience of communicating with older adults has been less effective, less respectful, less person centered, and perhaps more stressful than satisfying, why do you believe that is? Make a list of what you could do to increase satisfaction and lower stress.

- Do you know someone whom you believe communicates more effectively, more respectfully, and less stressfully with older adults than you? What is it that this person does differently than you? List the major differences and imagine how you could cultivate these skills, characteristics, or attitudes.

Using a scale of 1–10 (1 is lowest, 10 highest), rate the level of person-centered respect you demonstrate in your current communications with older adults.

What is one thing you could do that would help the older adults you serve to feel more seen, heard, and understood? Are there organizational barriers in place that might interfere with what you believe would be helpful?

Think about a healthcare provider with whom you have an effective, satisfying, respectful relationship. What is it specifically that makes this relationship effective, satisfying, and respectful? What does the provider do and say (or not do and not say) to earn your trust and respect? How does he or she encourage effective communication?

## MODEL OF AGING AND COMMUNICATION

This book embraces a bio-psycho-social model of aging that is also informed by Erick Erickson's stages of development theory. Erick Erikson (1902–1994) was "a German born US psychologist, preeminent personality theorist, and contributor to the field of ego psychology; known for his theory of life stages, Erickson's eight stages of development" (VandenBos, 2009, p. 469).

Focusing on how providers can communicate more effectively, more respectfully, and less stressfully with older adults, this book offers evidence-based suggestions grounded in a psychological model of communication heavily influenced by the person-centered perspective formulated by Carl Rogers. Carl Rogers (1902–1987) was a "US psychologist and originator of client centered therapy" (VandenBos, 2009, p. 475). Roger's person-centered approach—which views each person as a unique individual deserving of dignity and respect—was a key element of the humanistic psychology movement that evolved over the 1950s and 1960s.

The Rogerian approach—a model originally developed for psycho-therapists that encourages congruence, dignity, empathy, respect, and genuineness to facilitate authentic communication—has also proven useful for communication with older adults (Sheldon, 2004). Commonly referred to as client-centered or patient-centered care, a research review completed by deSilva (2014), found that person-centered care could result in increased client and provider satisfaction and improved health outcomes.

A major premise and recurring theme throughout this book is that the quality of the provider–older adult relationship can be improved and communication enhanced when providers do the following:

- Commit to using a person-centered approach to service delivery.
- Continue to develop their professional-level communication skills.
- Reduce inappropriate use of technical and professional jargon.
- Eliminate ageist attitudes and language.
- Understand how cultural differences and age-related physical, social, and psychological changes in the older adult can influence the communication process.

Providers who adopt the communication guidelines discussed throughout this book can expect to improve the overall communication experience, increase mutual respect and understanding, enhance accurate exchange of information, improve compliance with provider recommendations, positively impact outcomes, and often save time while lowering frustration and stress for the provider and the older adult.

## PLAIN TALK

Much of scientific and academic writing is dry, wordy, full of technical jargon, overly complex, difficult to understand, and—to be honest—boring. In contrast, this book was written using a *Plain Language* style. The Plain Language approach minimizes the use of professional jargon.

The goal is to be simple and direct without being too informal. Plain Language strives to be easy to read, understand, and use. Clear communication is a professional and ethical responsibility—whether written or spoken.

Plain Language is a growing, global movement whose mission is to reintroduce "plain talk" back into government, legal, scientific, and academic writing. The goal is to increase reader comprehension and reduce confusion by organizing information logically and writing in a manner that is focused on the needs of the reader http://centerforplainlanguage.org.

## AUTHOR'S EXPERIENCE: MY FIRST HOSPICE PATIENT

As a medical social worker, my first hospice patient was a feisty, 4′ 9″, 101-year-old woman. She spoke little during the early months of our visits, but in the weeks leading up to her death, she opened up and shared some of the challenges faced in growing older.

Retirement meant the loss of some of her financial security and the comfort of a daily routine. Changes in physical and mental health brought loss of agility, beauty, and energy. It also brought pain, loss of driving ability, loss of mobility, and some loss of independence.

Shortly before her death, she shared that the hardest part of living so long was outliving nearly every person she had ever known—family, spouse, friends, and acquaintances—everyone with the exception of her two sons (who at that time were nearing age 80). This was a woman who had lived through the introduction of the automobile, woman's rights, the electrification of planet earth, the birth of talking movies, World Wars I and II, nuclear energy, civil rights, the Vietnam war, and the invention of personal computers, the internet, and cell phones.

One afternoon, she called me to her bedside. With a barely audible voice, she pointed a trembling, bony, index finger at me, and said, "Tim, for the first few months after we met, I never really liked you much" (long pause) "but I want you to know something" (another long pause) "you're all right!" Those were the last words she spoke to me.

I don't know what changed her mind about how she felt about me. Maybe it was because I had shown her respect. When she spoke I paid attention. My words and actions communicated my belief that her agenda was more important than mine. There was no trying to tell her how she should or should not feel nor any attempt to get her to do anything she did not want to do. Week after week, I just kept showing up, letting her know I cared and was present if she felt like talking. I offered her person-centered, respect-based services—the topic and focus of this book.

## WORTH REMEMBERING

The motto below is from the mission statement of the Bombay Hospital in India. Substitute the word *patient* with *client, customer,* or *resident* to capture the essence of person-centered care.

> A patient is the most important part of our hospital. He is not an interruption to our work, he is the purpose of it. He is not an outsider in our hospital, he is a part of it. We're not doing him a favor by serving him, he is doing us a favor by giving us an opportunity to do so (Bombay Hospital).

Whether older adults are waiting in line at the pharmacy counter, reading a magazine in the reception area at the dentist, or walking down the hall of an assisted living facility, the message is the same—older adults are the most important part of your organization, the purpose for it, and the reason your profession exists. Be grateful. They are doing you the favor of giving you their business.

## CONCLUSION

Older adults are the fastest growing segment of the US and global population. This increase—related to the baby boom generation—is expected to impact most aspects of society over the next 20 years.

The quality of communication between service providers and older adults is important and can impact the service quality and resulting interactions. For service providers, communicating with older adults can be rewarding yet demanding and stressful.

A large percentage of older adults are dissatisfied with providers and cite the quality of the relationship as the main reason. Poor communication results from overuse of professional jargon and widespread ageist attitudes. Communication can be further impeded by the normal aging process, and by age-related physical, social, and psychological changes.

The position of this book is that communication is mutually interactive; it is interpersonal. Older adults are not objects to be spoken *at*, they are people to be spoken *with*. In every encounter, the older adult wants to be seen for who she or he is—a person, heard and listened to, respected, and appreciated. In each encounter, the older adult is listening, not only to the content of what is being communicated, but to how he or she is being treated (Greene & Burleson, 2003).

## LIST OF MAIN POINTS FOR PREVIEW AND REVIEW

- Clear communication is a professional and ethical responsibility.
- This book was written using a *Plain Language* style. The Plain Language approach minimizes the use of professional jargon.
- Older adults (individuals age 65 or older) are the fastest growing segment of the population in the United States and globally. This increase is expected to significantly impact most aspects of society and the related network of service providers.
- Growing numbers of older adults are voicing dissatisfaction with service providers. The main reasons cited are the poor quality of the provider–older adult relationships and unsatisfactory interpersonal communication.
- Unsatisfactory communication can impact the quality of services rendered as well as service outcomes.
- This chapter introduces five major causes of ineffective provider communication and argues for a person-centered, respect-based, Plain Language approach to communicating with older adults.
- By adopting the recommended communication guidelines, providers can often improve the overall communication experience, increase mutual respect and understanding, enhance accurate exchange of information, improve compliance with provider recommendations, positively impact outcomes, and save time while lowering frustration and stress for the provider and the older adult.
- In every encounter with providers, older adults want to be seen for who they are, listened to and heard, and respected and appreciated. Each wants to feel as if she or he matters enough for the provider to offer a few minutes of undivided attention.

• The provider's task is simple (yet frequently challenging)—keep the needs of the older adult as the central focus of service. See, hear, and interact with the individual as a unique person and not as a "patient," "client," or "customer."

**Provider Self-Test and/or Discussion Suggestions for Instructors**

**Discuss:** Why so many older adults feel dissatisfied with the quality of their provider relationships and how providers can reduce this dissatisfaction.

**Describe:** The five causes of older adult dissatisfaction.

**Explain:** The Plain Language/Plain Talk approach to communicating and how it differs from approaches that utilize a more formal, overly complex, jargon-based style.

**List:** Some of the costs of misunderstanding and miscommunication for the older adult, the provider, and the society.

**Contemplate:** Professional experience and recall recent experiences of communicating with older adults. Contemplate the main features of an effective, respectful, person-centered communication approach. Be able to tease out and distinguish the main differences of this approach from a less effective, disrespectful, ageist, provider-centered approach.

**Personal Reflection:** Identify personal areas of communication strength and list areas where improvement is desired.

## SELECT PROFESSIONAL JOURNALS

*Clinical Gerontologist*
*The Journal of Aging and Mental Health*
   http://www.routledgementalhealth.com/journals/details/0731-7115/
   Designed for counselors, nurses, physicians, psychologists, and social workers who address the issues of later life.
*Generations*
   http://www.asaging.org/generations-journal-american-society-aging
   In-depth research, practical applications, and valuable insight into the lives of older adults and those who work with them.
*Geriatric Nursing*
   http://www.gnjournal.com
   Specifically for nurses and nurse practitioners who work with older adults. Offers a comprehensive source for clinical information and management advice relating to the older adult care.

*Journal of Aging Studies*
  http://www.journals.elsevier.com/journal-of-aging-studies/
  Features scholarly papers offering challenging interpretations of existing
  theory and empirical work.
*Journal of Applied Gerontology*
  http://jag.sagepub.com/
  Comprehensive coverage of all areas of gerontological practice and pol-
  icy, such as caregiving, exercise, death and dying, ethnicity and aging,
  technology and care, long-term care, mental health, and sexuality.
*Journal of Cross-Cultural Gerontology*
  http://link.springer.com/journal/10823
  Applied approaches, research findings, and theoretical issues that deal
  with non-Western populations.
*Journal of Gerontological Nursing*
  http://www.healio.com/nursing/journals/jgn
  Original articles on the practice of gerontological nursing across the
  continuum of care in a variety of healthcare settings.
*Journal of Gerontological Social Work*
  http://www.tandfonline.com/action/journalInformation?show=aims
  Scope&journalCode=wger20#.VHNm45XF-zQ
  Devoted to social work administration, consultation, practice, and theory in the field of aging.
*Journal of Social Work in End-of-Life & Palliative Care*
  http://www.tandfonline.com/toc/wswe20/current#.VHNnQJXF-zQ
  Original articles and research that explore issues crucial to individuals
  with serious, life-threatening, and life-limiting illness and their families
  across the life span.
*Journal of the American Geriatrics Society*
  http://geriatricscareonline.org/ProductAbstract/journal-of-the-americ
  an-geriatrics-society/J001
  Research and information about common diseases and disorders of
  older adults.
*Journal of Women & Aging*
  http://www.tandfonline.com/toc/wjwa20/current#.VHNnvZXF-zQ
  Provides administrators, educators, practitioners, and researchers with a
  comprehensive guide to the unique challenges facing older women.
*Psychology and Aging*
  http://www.apa.org/pubs/journals/pag/index.aspx
  Original articles on adult development and aging.

*The Gerontologist*
http://gerontologist.oxfordjournals.org/
A multidisciplinary perspective on human aging published by The
Gerontological Society of America.

## WEB RESOURCES

**Aging**
American Psychological Association: Office on Aging
  http://www.apa.org/pi/aging/index.aspx
American Society on Aging
  www.asaging.org
Gero Central
  http://gerocentral.org
Global Aging Research Network
  http://www.garn-network.org/index.php
National Academy on an Aging Society
  www.agingsociety.org/agingsociety/links/index.html
The Gerontological Society of America
  www.geron.org
World Health Organization
  http://www.who.int/topics/ageing/en/

**Person-Centered Care**
Institute for Person-Centered Care
  http://ubipcc.com/

**Plain Language Resources**
  http://centerforplainlanguage.org
  http://www.nih.gov/clearcommunication/plainlanguage/index.htm
  http://www.plainlanguage.gov/whatisPL/

## REFERENCES

Bombay Hospital. http://www.bombayhospital.com.
Centers for Disease Control and Prevention. (2014). http://www.cdc.gov/niosh/topics/healthcare/.
Charcot, J. (1983). *Chanting the universe: Hawaiian religious culture*. Honolulu, HI: Emphasis International.
de Silva, D. (2014). *Helping measure person-centred care: A review of evidence about commonly used approaches and tools used to help measure person-centred care*. London, UK: The Health Foundation.
Dossey, L. (2011). *Healing words*. San Francisco, CA: Harper Collins.

Drench, M. E., Noonan, A. C., Sharby, N., & Ventura, S. H. (2012). *Psychosocial aspects of health care*. New York: Pearson.

Gerontology News. (2014). *Gerontological society of America*.

Greene, J. O., & Burleson, B. R. (Eds.). (2003). *Handbook of communication and social interaction skills*. Mahwah, NJ: Lawrence Erlbaum Associates, Inc.

Hart, V. A. (2010). *Patient-provider communications: Caring to listen*. Sudbury, MA: Jones and Bartlett Publishers.

James, J. T. (2013). A new evidence-based estimate of patient harms associated with hospital care. *Journal of Patient Safety, 9*(3), 122–128.

Knapp, M. L., & Daly, J. A. (Eds.). (2011). *The sage handbook of interpersonal communication*.

Mish, F. C. (Ed.). (2009). *Merriam-Webster's collegiate dictionary*. Springfield, MS: Merriam-Webster, Inc.

Pew Social Trends. http://www.pewsocialtrends.org.

Phelps, K., & Hassed, C. (2012). *Communication with patients*. Kindle Edition. Chatswood, NSW: Elsevier (Australia).

Robnett, R. H., & Chop, W. C. (2010). *Gerontology for healthcare professionals*. Sudbury, MA: Jones and Bartlett Publishers.

Sheldon, L. K. (2004). *Communication for nurses: Talking with patients*. Thorofare, NJ: Slack, Inc.

Tamparo, C. D., & Lindh, W. Q. (2008). *Therapeutic communications for healthcare*. Clifton Park, New York: Thompson Delmar Learning.

United States Census Bureau. (2011). https://www.census.gov/newsroom/releases/archives/facts_for_features_special_editions/cb11-ff08.html.

United States Department of Health and Human Services. (2013). http://www.hhs.gov/.

VandenBos, G. R. (2009). *College dictionary of psychology*. Washington, DC: American Psychological Association.

Williams, A., & Nussbaum, J. F. (2001). *Intergenerational communication across the lifespan*. Mahwah, NJ: Lawrence Erlbaum Associates.

World Healthcare Organization. (2014). http://www.who.int/topics/ageing/en/.

CHAPTER 2

# How to Learn and Implement the Person-Centered Approach to Communication

*The only person who is educated is the one who has learned how to learn and change.*

*Carl Rogers*

**Core Question**: How can providers learn and implement the person-centered approach to interpersonal communication?

**Keywords**: Conscious competence; Conscious incompetence; Implementation science; Mindfulness; Non-maleficence; Person-centered; Provider-centered; SMART goals; Unconscious competence; Unconscious incompetence; Worldview.

## INTRODUCTION—THE CORE PROBLEM AND FIVE KEY RECOMMENDATIONS

Chapter 1 pointed out that many older adults feel dissatisfied with their current service provider relationships. This dissatisfaction stems primarily from problematic provider–older adult interpersonal communication. To increase understanding of how providers can effectively and respectfully communicate with older adults, five key recommendations were listed—core suggestions that are interwoven and emphasized throughout this book.

1. Complete additional training on how to communicate with older adults.
2. Learn and implement a person-centered communication approach.
3. Embrace a "plain talk" style when communicating with older adults and reduce inappropriate use of confusing professional jargon.
4. Identify, reduce, and eliminate ageist attitudes and language.
5. Understand how the interpersonal communication process can be impacted by cultural differences and by age-related physical, social, and psychological changes often experienced by older adults.

*Person-Centered Communication with Older Adults*
http://dx.doi.org/10.1016/B978-0-12-420132-3.00002-7

This chapter begins with the discussion of the first recommendation: Complete additional training on how to communicate with older adults. The remaining recommendations will be explored in later chapters.

Chapter 1 presented an overview of "what" providers could expect to learn from this book. This chapter offers evidence-based suggestions for "how" to learn the what. This chapter presents a systematic learning strategy for approaching the information, knowledge, and practices contained in the rest of the book—a unique approach designed to encourage professional growth, learning, and skill building. Employing these strategies, practical planning suggestions, goal-setting techniques, and implementation methods should prove helpful in developing a person-centered approach to communicating. Among other things, providers will be shown the following:

- The characteristics of competent communicators and ways to emulate them.
- How to recognize, analyze, and modify stimulus/response patterns associated with interpersonal communication using imaginary interactions?
- How to identify current personal strengths and target areas needing improvement using a four-stage model for mastering new learning and skill?
- How to develop a personal professional growth plan?

Providers who carefully study the information provided, who compare the case examples with their own experience, who wrestle with the conceptual material, who invest the effort necessary to identify their professional communication strengths and weaknesses, who complete the suggested exercises, and who consistently apply what is learned from this in their daily professional arena will almost certainly notice constructive changes–changes in personal worldview, and more importantly, changes in the quality of interactions with older adults.

## FIRST—DO NO HARM

Providers who work with older adults have an ethical responsibility to "first, do no harm." The principle of non-harm or non-maleficence is one of the foundational precepts of healthcare bioethics—part of the Hippocratic Oath historically taken by physicians and other healthcare professionals. Adopting a person-centered versus provider-centered approach to communication with older adults is one way to help reduce risk of unintentionally inflicting harm.

*You can't die tonight, honey, I need to get paid for a full shift!*

The preceding quote was an actual comment directed to a 91-year-old, bed-ridden patient by an employee of a skilled-care nursing facility. The employee's words may have been spoken in jest, but their disrespectful effect on the patient was no laughing matter.

The incident was reported to the facility director who also failed to see the humor in this remark. She reminded the now ex-employee that words can help or harm, and all members of the healthcare network—from aides to physicians—share a responsibility to protect the patient to "first, do no harm." This example illustrates how communication can be defined more by what the listener hears than by what the speaker intended. It is vital for providers to develop a person-centered approach to communication grounded in a knowledgeable and respectful view of the aging process and of older adults.

## THE IMPORTANCE OF WORLDVIEW

Another prime objective of this chapter is to invite providers to cultivate a perspective or worldview of aging and older adults that fosters a more respectful, person-centered style of communication. The provider is encouraged to revise any views that might foster ageist attitudes and language, reduce use of professional jargon when interacting with older adults, and to adopt a person-centered perspective of service delivery as opposed to the often observed provider-centered approach.

Each provider's personal view influences his or her communication process. This view can be purposefully modified to support a more person-centered perspective.

## HOW PERSONAL VIEW INFLUENCES THE COMMUNICATION PROCESS

A worldview is a set of assumptions, beliefs, and interpreted experiences that informs and influences (among other things) attitudes and understanding of aging, older persons, and the provider–older adult interpersonal communication process. This view is created by the human brain as it attempts to identify, categorize, explain, and interpret daily experiences, derive meaning from them, reduce fear of the unknown and unexplained, and predict the probable future (Feinstein & Krippner, 2006).

The brain's creation of a personal worldview is accomplished through a complex process that can be thought of as "connecting the dots" and by generating what could be conceived as a personal internal narrative (or story). This narrative story functions as an individual's view of the world. It emerges from the neural activities of the brain as it processes information into premises to arrive at meaning and conclusions.

Feinstein and Krippner (2006) suggest these personal stories (or worldviews) are a type of infrastructure that function to inform and guide the individual. This infrastructure is thought to consist of beliefs, feelings, and rules that operate at a mostly preconscious level outside of everyday, normal wakeful awareness. Although this process is operational primarily at a preconscious level, conscious interpretation of the meaning of experience can help shape and modify an existing view—an important consideration for providers determined to adopt a more person-centered perspective.

## PURPOSEFUL MODIFICATION OF WORLDVIEW

A worldview is malleable and subject to modification, based on new learning and experience (Feinstein & Krippner, 2006). During the natural process of human maturation, the veracity of personal narratives or worldviews are often challenged, and the need for revision is frequent. Some views are challenged from biological, emotional, and mental growth. Others are challenged by exposure to new information, concepts, people, and specific circumstances that contradict the underlying premises of the stories.

Newburg (2006) suggests these personal stories—that people such as providers create—are organized explanations created by a brain that seeks to categorize and connect together new experiences with previous memories, beliefs, needs, and fears. This weaving process creates a preconscious narration that organizes perceptions and feelings, establishes their meaning, and influences thoughts, values, ethics, decisions, and behaviors.

These internal narratives seem to function as "connecting threads" that weave personal experience and life events together to form a story that helps explain "why things are the way they are." This worldview helps each individual make sense of his or her world. Harmon (1988) believes these stories are deeply ingrained assumptions and generalizations that influence understanding and influence behavior.

## NARRATIVE STORIES INFLUENCE PHYSIOLOGY

An individual's worldview can shape his or her interpretations of experience and thoughts, and—from the choices made—can influence behavior. These stories can be compared to a lens that colors perception. They seem to function in a manner similar to a template that provides a ready-made set of assumptions, tenants, expectations, and conclusions—all of which the brain assumes to be accurate and true.

## HOW NARRATIVE STORIES CAN IMPACT PHYSIOLOGY

Freeman and Lawlis (2001) describe the underlying mechanisms by which mental or narrative interpretation can impact physiology. Briefly, the three systems involved in this communication process are the nervous system, endocrine system, and immune system. These three systems communicate by using two pathways: the sympathetic-adrenal-medullary axis and the hypothalamic-pituitary-adrenal cortex axis. These pathways, in turn, use various messenger molecules to influence physiology.

Dawson (2007) goes into considerable detail explaining how the human body responds to thought and feeling. For example, he suggests there are over 1400 chemical reactions and over 30 hormones and neurotransmitters that can shift in response to perceived stressful stimuli. This overly simplified explanation outlines the process by which thoughts influence the body. The related topic of the stress-response will be discussed in much greater detail in a later chapter.

In summary, as events are experienced, an individual categorizes and assigns meaning to them. The specific category or meaning assigned can trigger which preconscious story (worldview) and script is activated and, as a result, which biochemicals are released into the body. So, the next time an older adult customer seems a little confused, or perhaps talks a bit too much, or maybe walks a little too slowly, remember that interpretation matters!

The following exercise is designed to demonstrate how stimulus/response patterns act as causative links in the chain of communication and to show how the interpretation an individual gives to an interaction can play a significant role in how he or she responds.

---

### Exercise 1: The Mother-in-Law and the Pharmacy Technician— Interpretation Matters!

**Learning Objectives:**

1. Improve ability to recognize, analyze, and modify stimulus/response patterns associated with interpersonal communication.
2. Practice modifying stimulus/response patterns using the technique of imaginary interactions (note: this exercise utilizes the technique of imaginary encounters and interactions—a highly beneficial process— that will be discussed in much more detail in a later chapter).

**Instructions:**

1. Read the following true story from start to finish.
2. Re-read the story a second time, but this time do so from the point of view of the mother-in-law. Imagine you are the mother-in-law.
3. Re-read the story for a third time, but this time do so from the point of view of the pharmacy technician. Imagine you are the pharmacy technician (tech).

*I was at the pharmacy with my mother-in-law. We waited in line with the rest of the customers, and when it was our turn, we stepped up to the counter. The pharmacy tech smiled, started processing the prescription, and then asked my mother-in-law a question. She became confused and started looking through her purse nervously. With a sigh, the tech looked at me as if to imply I should answer his question for her. Sensing his impatience, I tried to help her answer the question, but by now, she was feeling embarrassed—like she was wasting everyone's time—and moved to the side of the counter so the tech could help someone else. The tech then remarked that he could not help anyone else because he had already started with my mother-in-law. He then rudely said to me, "Can't you just answer this for her?" I told him no, I could not, that it was something she'd be able to figure out within a minute or so. At this point, my mother-in-law felt flustered and said, "Just forget it," and she withdrew her medication purchase. In silence, we walked back to our car and left. On the way back to her apartment, my mother-in-law sat in the car sobbing.*

*After a few minutes—when she was able to talk—she told me, "I'm never going back there again!"*

To complete this exercise, re-read the story for a fourth and final time, maintaining the perspective of the pharmacy tech. Contemplate the details of the patterns of communication that occurred from a stimulus/response perspective. Example: The pharmacy tech did/said "X" (a stimulus) which led the mother-in-law to say/do "Y" (a response). Use imagination to change whatever details of the story are necessary to create a completed purchase and a satisfied customer who felt respected.

In other words, mentally modify the pattern of stimulus/response until the desired outcome of a "happy ending" is achieved. This widely used technique is a form of *behavioral rehearsal*—a term used to "describe a specific procedure which aims to replace deficient or inadequate social or interpersonal responses by efficient and effective behavioral patterns" (Bellack & Hersen, 1985, p. 22).

When this exercise is performed in a small group, it is often valuable for participants to share and discuss what they believe could have been said or done differently to create a more desirable outcome.

## SIGNIFICANCE OF MENTAL INTERPRETATION IN FORMING WORLDVIEW

With reference to the story used in Exercise 1, the pharmacy tech acted impatiently, demonstrated less than stellar customer service, and communicated in a disrespectful manner. His actions upset the daughter-in-law, hurt the feelings of the mother-in-law, cost him a sale, and lost him a lifetime customer.

The mother-in-law's current monthly prescription costs are $187. She will probably need to be on these medications for the remainder of her life. If she lives another five years, and the costs remain the same, the total amount of revenue this pharmacy will lose due to the actions of this single unsatisfactory interaction is $11,220. This figure does not include any purchases that may have come from the daughter-in-law.

The specific thoughts and feelings that led the pharmacy tech to respond in this manner are unknown. What can be surmised is that this provider was operating from a particular worldview associated with and triggered by his interpretation of circumstances—perhaps a view more provider-centered than person-centered. The details, logic, and conclusions of his preconscious story provided a script-like rationale for his response.

It can also be surmised that if the pharmacy tech had come to a different interpretation (or conclusion) about this circumstance, a different story might have been accessed (or triggered) that could have led to a different response. To clarify, assume there were a dozen customers standing in line. Speculate the provider was looking at these customer faces and imagining they were in a hurry—feeling impatient because he was taking too long serving the mother-in-law. He felt pressured. Assume he concluded, "This old lady is talking and moving way too slowly."

If these speculations are accurate, then a particular story (or script) was activated at the preconscious level of awareness, a story that, for whatever reasons, made him feel impatient and, thus, triggered the stress-response— a topic that will explored in detail in a later chapter. The point is this: All of the provider's responses were triggered by his interpretation of the current circumstances—his conclusion about what it meant. But, what if he had interpreted this situation differently? What if he had come to an alternative conclusion—triggered an alternative narrative story? Chances are his response would have also been different.

Kabat-Zinn (1990) provides detailed information describing how mental interpretations of a specific circumstance can alter and impact experience. Apparently, the level of psychological comfort or discomfort experienced from exposure to events depends, at least in part, on the mental interpretations given to these events. If this is accurate, then how a provider interprets, judges, or explains his or her experiences can directly influence physiology and levels of emotional comfort or discomfort.

## OVERALL APPROACH FOR LEARNING TO IMPROVE COMMUNICATION

Understanding that a provider's response to an encounter with an older adult is influenced by the provider's interpretation of that interaction is an important realization and underscores the importance of worldview. It is a helpful first step, but much more is needed.

At this early stage of the learning process, it is useful to define and embrace an overall approach to the process of knowledge and skill acquisition—a key objective of this chapter. Spitzberg and Cupach (1984) identified three general requirements that can be adapted for providers seeking to improve communication skills:

1. Motivation: The provider must desire to improve his or her ability to successfully communicate with older adults.
2. Knowledge: The provider should develop an understanding of the aging process and of the age-related physical, emotional, and mental changes commonly experienced in this population that can impact interpersonal communication.
3. Skills: The provider must develop the skill-set necessary to competently and successfully communicate with older adults.

This three-step model is used extensively throughout this book as a means of organizing information. As readers study, explore, discuss and implement the materials provided in each chapter, they will cycle and recycle through these same three steps—motivation, knowledge acquisition, and skill building. This should enhance the learning experience.

## SHAPING WORLDVIEW

In the previous chapter, providers were encouraged to reflect on personal professional experience related to communicating with older adults. This review included listing attitudes, behaviors, and skills believed to contribute to successful communication.

Providers were asked to identify an individual who demonstrates the ability to communicate with older adults in an effective, respectful, person-centered manner—a person who could serve as a mental role model. Finally, providers were asked to recall a satisfying professional relationship that they have with a healthcare provider—someone who is a competent communicator—and then to think about what aspects of the relationship and of that individual's skill set contribute to the favorable impression and experience. These types of contemplative activities help influence and shape worldview.

## IMPLEMENTATION SCIENCE

Important breakthrough innovations are historically frequent. Some have the potential to enhance quality of life and increase life expectancy. The process of translating potential improvements into actual improvements is complex and influenced by the various stakeholders involved—regulatory bodies, politicians, providers, patients, etc. At the level of the collective provider network, this struggle falls under the umbrella of *implementation science*.

Implementation science focuses on how innovative research findings are disseminated and implemented at the level of practice (Demiris, Oliver, Capurro, & Wittenberg-Lyles, 2014). This formalized process—known as the implementation and dissemination process or I&D—is the focus of this chapter.

## PROVIDER MOTIVATION TO IMPROVE COMMUNICATION SKILLS

A provider's motivation to learn and implement improved communication skills can stem from internal and/or external sources. Providers who completed the review of personal professional experience suggested in Chapter 1, may have already identified reasons for wanting to improve communication skills. These reasons might relate to how the provider could benefit and/or how the older adult, agency, or organization could benefit from improved interpersonal communication.

Motivation to improve communication skills also stems from external sources. A provider could have received feedback from an older adult, a colleague, or supervisor that made it clear improvements were needed. The provider may have been exposed to new information from a book, newspaper, professional journal article, or something from the Internet or TV that led to new insights, knowledge, or understanding.

Whether internal, external, or a combination of both, it is necessary for each provider to identify his or her personal motivations for wanting to improve the ability to communicate with older adults. During the sometimes lengthy process of professional knowledge building and skill acquisition, it can be reenergizing and renewing to remind oneself why such improvements are important.

## THE NEXT STEPS

To improve the provider–older adult interpersonal communication process, providers need to build a strong knowledge base and begin development of foundational skills. Recommendations for achieving this include the following:
- Examine personal motivations for wanting to complete additional communication training.
- Reflect on current strengths and weakness.
- Adopt an overall approach to the process of knowledge building and skill acquisition.
- Cultivate a worldview of the aging process and of older adults that fosters a respectful, person–centered style of communication.

- Practice analyzing the stimulus/response patterns of communication and modifying these patterns using the technique of imaginary interactions.
- List and reflect upon the major qualities and characteristics of competent communicators.
- Identify someone that can be used as a mental role model.
- Recall a personally satisfying professional relationship with a provider. List the qualities and skills this person possesses that demonstrate his or her communication skills.

After completion of the above, the next step is to formulate a professional growth plan. When completed, this plan can serve as a roadmap outlining how additional knowledge about the aging process and older adults will be acquired and which specific communication skills require further personal development.

## PROVIDERS AS EFFECTIVE COMMUNICATORS

The literature is replete with lists of characteristics of providers considered to be effective communicators (Phelps & Hassed, 2012). Frequently cited characteristics include the following:

- Provider is more person-centered than provider-centered (focused on the older adult vs focused on self).
- Provider is more person-focused than problem-focused (focused first on the person and second on the problem).
- Provider demonstrates a high degree of compassionate commitment to the older adult.
- Provider displays a humanistic approach to relationships as opposed to a technological orientation.
- Provider style is often compared to that of the old-fashioned family doctor.
- Provider evinces concern, congruence, empathy, genuineness, respect, and unconditional positive regard for older adult.
- Provider is attentive, listens mindfully, and minimizes multitasking.

### Exercise 2: Self-Rating of Person-Centered Characteristics
**Learning Objective**: Increase personal awareness of current person-centered skill set.

#### Instructions:
**1.** Re-read the list of characteristics of competent, person-centered communicators in the previous section.

2. Using a 1 to 5 Likert scale, rate the current skill level with respect to each statement above: 1 = mostly inaccurate and untrue; 5 = mostly accurate and true.

3. After completion of self-assessment, reflect on the pattern of your ratings. Consider establishing SMART goals for any areas in need of improvement. For establishing clear goals, many professionals use an approach commonly referred to as the SMART process. SMART is an acronym that refers to goals that are specific, measurable, achievable, realistic, and timely.

## CLEAR INTENTIONS LEAD TO CLEAR RESULTS

The process of learning something new or improving current knowledge or skills is assisted by clearly defined intentions or objectives. If it is accurate to state that clear intentions often lead to clear results, then it is accurate to state that vague intentions frequently lead to vague results. Defining learning intentions by creating specific, well-formed goals helps providers develop a professional growth plan that is efficient and effective.

Each provider is encouraged to develop a personal professional growth plan. As previously described, SMART is an acronym that stands for specific, measurable, achievable, relevant, and time framed (Doran, 1981). Use of the SMART process can assist with translating theory into practice.

**S**—Specific: Select a specific goal(s). This means the provider decides what he or she specifically wants to accomplish. Although it might be preferable to complete study of this book before completing the SMART goal process, even at this early stage, it could prove helpful to formulate 1–2 preliminary goals. Examples are "Learn how to form a respectful professional relationship with an older adult" or "Learn the nuts-and-bolts of the person-centered communication approach." During the process of formulating goals, it is often helpful to imagine the goal has already been achieved, and then contemplate how this achievement enhanced the ability to communicate more effectively and satisfactorily with older adults. Imagining comments that colleagues might make once this goal has been achieved can also be helpful. Finally, consider what achieving this goal would mean personally. The chapter that focuses on mental imagery contains many useful methods to help accomplish this.

**M**—Measurable: This step in the goal-setting process is focused on measuring learning or improvement. Example: If the goal was to gain knowledge about how age-related hearing changes can impact the interpersonal communication process, how could improvement be measured or demonstrated? A well-formed SMART goal describes what the baseline level of knowledge or skill was before new learning occurred and includes a way of measuring or demonstrating that a change in baseline occurred. Tests, essays, group discussion, supervisory or peer observations, and customer or client feedback are some of the ways new learning or improvement in skills could be demonstrated.

**A**—Achievable: Given current circumstances, motivation, time, and available resources, is this goal achievable? After careful reflection, a short, honest answer is best.

**R**—Relevant: What is important about gaining additional knowledge about how age-related hearing changes can impact the interpersonal communication process? Justify your goal to yourself. Why is achieving this goal important? How will it benefit you or satisfy some specific need?

**T**—Time framed: When will this goal be achieved? Setting realistic deadlines are important.

In summary, contemplate desirable learning or improvement objectives. Choose what seems important, needed, beneficial, and/or something that satisfies a specific need. Create SMART goals for help in achieving objectives. Once the SMART goal-setting process has been completed and related learning and/or training is underway, each provider will progress from ignorance to mastery as described in the four stages of learning model explained in the next section.

## FOUR-STAGE MODEL OF MASTERING NEW LEARNING AND/OR SKILLS

Each provider will have some level of communication knowledge and related skill sets already in place. Some areas may be highly developed, some moderately so, and others lacking or in need of significant improvement. Exercise 2: *Self-rating of Person-centered Characteristics* was designed to help providers begin to identify areas where improvement might be needed.

No matter which goals or skills were selected for improvement, the acquisition and mastery of any new knowledge or skill will typically pass through four well-recognized phases. This four-stage model provides a useful outline of the journey experienced when undertaking new learning.

This new knowledge or skill could be anything from learning to drive a car, learning to play a musical instrument, to becoming more person-centered.

Learning, improving, and eventual mastery of new knowledge or skills follow a similar path and trajectory of development. Example: Using this model, a provider learning how to be more person-centered would pass through—or would have already passed through—one or more of the following four conceptual stages:

Stage 1: *Unconscious Incompetence.* In this first stage of learning, the provider has virtually no awareness of the topic or the specific skills involved in developing a person-centered approach to communication. This stage can be compared to getting behind the wheel of car for the very first time in preparation for learning to drive. At this stage, the learner is often ignorant of what he or she does not yet know, will be expected to know, and may one day actually know. He or she may not be sure of what questions to ask, where to begin learning, or how to organize the overall learning experience. This initial stage is typically transcended quickly from exposure to new information, reflection on rationale and mutual benefits for adopting the new approach, listening to explanations, role-playing and viewing demonstrations, and via receiving feedback from older adults, supervisors, and/or peers. With persistent and adequate motivation, repeated exposure to the information, appropriate personal reflection, feedback, and practice, the provider progresses to the second stage of learning.

Stage 2: *Conscious Incompetence.* If the learning process is continued, the provider begins to understand what remains unknown and how much remains to be learned. Mentally recalling past unsatisfactory interactions with older adults, reflecting on the root causes of the dissatisfaction, and then contemplating what could have been done differently to produce a more desirable outcome aids in bringing the underlying involved processes and skills to conscious awareness. Exercise 1—presented earlier in this chapter—is an example of using this mental process for expanding awareness. Once brought to conscious awareness, the learner begins to understand what to pay attention to, to realize what it is he or she does not yet know or understand, and to better sense the overall direction of the process of learning or skill acquisition. With adequate and persistent motivation, repeated practice of person-centered concepts in the service arena, and continued feedback and personal reflection, the provider progresses to the third stage of learning.

Stage 3: *Conscious Competence.* This is the stage where the provider can purposely adopt a person-centered approach to communicating. At this step in developing mastery, the psychological state of mind and skills involved in applying the person-centered approach are consciously and purposefully evoked. Although the provider clearly understands the underlying principles and techniques for utilizing a person-centered approach, they are not yet automatic and using them may feel a bit awkward or mechanical. With enough desire and persistence, with regular and continued use in the service arena over a long period of time, and with occasional feedback from older adults, colleagues, and/or supervisors, technical proficiency continues to develop. Eventually, some will progress to the fourth and final stage of learning—mastery.

Stage 4: *Unconscious Competence.* This is the level of the expert where knowledge and skills are available automatically. This is the stage where the provider can apply the knowledge and skills when and where needed without conscious effort. They flow automatically out of the depths of hard-earned experience and deep knowing. Although this is not the end of learning—because there is no end to learning—it is, to use a martial arts concept, the black-belt level where mastery begins. In many ways, a provider will always be a learner, but at this level, he or she can also be considered a role model and teacher.

## BARRIERS TO IMPROVING COMMUNICATION WITH OLDER ADULTS

Most providers would probably welcome the opportunity to complete additional training designed to improve their ability to communicate more effectively with older adults. Unfortunately, barriers often exist that make it difficult to complete such training.

Many providers struggle with the scheduling and time-management demands that frequently accompany large patient, client, or resident caseloads. Customer lines can be long, schedules tight, and service delivery often occurs in a complex professional environment, top-heavy with regulatory guidelines and documentation requirements. Free time for continuing professional education can often feel scarce.

The challenge to stay informed and up-to-date can be a constant struggle for the individual provider and for the collective network of service providers. Demiris et al. (2014) point out, "There has been a near-continuous stream of breakthrough innovations in virtually every area of health care" (p. 163). Yet, the common workplace atmosphere often leaves the provider with little time for continuing education—to keep abreast of advances in their field.

Even with the highest intentions and the best professional growth plan in place, providers still often face barriers to the acquisition of person-centered communication skills. Healthcare clinicians may lack experience with some of the aspects and skills of person-centered communication, such as the following:

1. Mindfulness: purposefully paying attention, in the present moment, nonjudgmentally (Kabat-Zinn, 1990).
2. Nonjudgmental listening: listening to the older adult without judging.
3. Asking open-ended questions: questions that cannot be answered with a "yes" or "no," nor with a specific, single piece of information.
4. Sharing power and decision-making: a collaborative process where responsibility for decision-making is shared between older adults and providers.

Instead of practicing these four characteristics of person-centered communication, medically oriented clinicians are often more comfortable operating from within a provider-centered model—relying on use of close-ended questions, controlling the interaction, reporting findings, and making recommendations (Phelps & Hassed, 2012).

## CONCLUSION

The systematic approach to achieving professional growth and associated learning strategies described in this chapter was designed to be used as a method for implementing the information, knowledge, and practices contained in the rest of the book. Employing these methods should prove helpful in developing a person-centered approach to communicating with older adults.

## LIST OF MAIN POINTS FOR PREVIEW AND REVIEW

• A systematic learning and implementation strategy can aid the provider in acquiring the knowledge and skills associated with the person-centered communication approach.
• Providers who work with older adults have an ethical responsibility to "first, do no harm."

- Adopting a person-centered approach is one way to help reduce risk of unintentionally inflicting harm.
- A worldview is a set of assumptions, beliefs, and interpreted experiences that informs and influences (among other things) attitudes and understanding of aging, older persons, and the provider–older adult interpersonal communication process. Providers can purposefully cultivate a perspective or worldview of aging and older adults that fosters a more respectful, person-centered style of communication, reduces unnecessary use of professional jargon, and eliminates ageist attitudes and language.
- The literature is replete with lists of characteristics of providers considered to be effective communicators. Frequently cited characteristics include more person-centered than provider-centered; more person-focused than problem-focused; a high degree of compassionate commitment to older adults; displays a humanistic approach to relationships as opposed to a technological orientation; often compared to that of the old-fashioned family doctor; evinces concern, congruence, empathy, genuineness, respect, and unconditional positive regard for older adult; and is attentive, listens mindfully, and minimizes multitasking.
- Providers can develop a personal professional growth plan based on the concept of creating SMART goals. SMART is an acronym that stands for specific, measurable, achievable, relevant, and time framed.
- When completed, a personal growth plan can serve as a roadmap outlining how additional knowledge about the aging process and older adults will be acquired and which specific communication skills require further personal development.
- The acquisition and mastery of any new knowledge or skill will typically pass through four well-recognized phases: unconscious incompetence, conscious incompetence, conscious competence, and unconscious competence.
- The systematic approach to achieving professional growth and associated learning strategies described in this chapter were designed to be used as a method for implementing the information, knowledge, and practices contained in the rest of the book. Employing these methods should prove helpful in developing a person-centered approach to communicating with older adults.

**Provider Self-Test and/or Discussion Suggestions for Instructors**

**Personal Reflection:** Reflect on the principle of *Primum non nocere*, a Latin phrase that means "first, do no harm" and how it relates to communicating with older adults.

**Compare and Contrast:** Compare and contrast characteristics of a person-centered style of communicating with a provider-centered approach.

**Discuss:** Discuss how a provider's worldview can influence perspective on the aging process, older adults, and interpersonal communication with older adults. Share details of how personal worldview can be consciously shaped to help foster a respectful, person-centered approach to service delivery.

**Speculate:** Using the case example provided in Exercise 1: *The mother-in-law and the pharmacy tech*, explore the role worldview played in this interaction. Using analysis of stimulus/response patterns, talk about what the pharmacy tech could have said and done differently to produce a more desirable outcome.

**Contemplate Professional Experience:** Reflect on how completion of a professional growth plan that includes SMART goals can guide and assist with the process of knowledge and skill acquisition. Consider how the *Four-phases of Learning* model can help identify the current level of knowledge and skill acquisition and suggest the next step needed for continued development.

# REFERENCES

Bellack, A. S., & Hersen, M. (1985). *Dictionary of behavior therapy techniques*. Elmsford, NY: Pergamon Press.

Dawson, C. (2007). *The genie in your genes*. Santa Rosa, CA: Elite Books.

Demiris, G., Oliver, D. P., Capurro, D., & Wittenberg-Lyles, E. (2014). Implementation science: implications for intervention research in hospice and palliative care. *The Gerontologist, 54*(2), 163–171.

Doran, G. T. (1981). There's a S.M.A.R.T. way to write management's goals and objectives. *Management Review, 70*(11), 35–36.

Feinstein, D., & Krippner, S. (2006). *The mythic path*. Santa Rosa, CA: Energy Psychology Press.

Freeman, L. W., & Lawlis, G. F. (2001). *Mosby's complementary and alternative medicine: A research-based approach*. St. Louis, MO: Mosby.

Harmon, W. (1988). *Global mind change*. San Francisco, CA: Warner Books.

Kabat-Zinn. (1990). *Full catastrophe living: Using the wisdom of your body and mind to face stress, pain, and illness*. New York, NY: Bantam Dell.

Newburg, A. (2006). *Why we believe what we believe*. New York, NY: Free Press.

Phelps, K., & Hassed, C. (2012). *Communication with patients*. Kindle Edition. Chatswood, NSW: Elsevier, Australia.

Spitzberg, B. H., & Cupach, W. R. (1984). *Interpersonal communication competence*. Beverly Hills, CA: Sage.

CHAPTER 3

# The Professional Relationship: The Foundation of Person-Centered Communication

*The meeting of two personalities is like the contact of two chemical substances: if there is any reaction, both are transformed.*

C.G. Jung

**Core Question**: How can a provider develop a respectful, person-centered relationship with an older adult?

**Keywords:** Deep listening; Elderspeak; Mindfulness; Mirroring; Multi-tasking; Person centered; Provider relationship; Rapport.

## INTRODUCTION: THE NEXT MOST IMPORTANT STEP

Many older adults are dissatisfied with the services rendered by their providers. This dissatisfaction is rooted in frustration about the quality of interpersonal communication. To address this core concern, Chapter 1 recommended providers to adopt a respect-based, person-centered, plain-language approach to communicating with older adults. Chapter 2 discussed systematic implementation methods that can help maximize professional growth, accelerate learning, and assist with the acquisition of person-centered communication skills.

The principle of non-malfeasance was introduced—a core concept emphasized throughout this book. This chapter discusses the next step—and possibly the most important step—how to establish a rapport-based professional relationship with an older adult.

## COMMUNICATION OCCURS WITHIN A RELATIONSHIP

Whether an interaction occurs at a pharmacy counter, in the hallway of an assisted living facility, or in a physician's examination room, communication between a provider and an older adult takes place within a professional relationship. Numerous studies have been conducted that focused on exploring communication styles and interactions between patients and health

*Person-Centered Communication with Older Adults*
http://dx.doi.org/10.1016/B978-0-12-420132-3.00003-9
**37**

professionals (de Silva, 2014). One common finding: Communication with an older adult does not occur in a vacuum. It occurs within a relationship, and effective communication is a learnable skill (Phelps & Hassed, 2012).

Professional relationships develop over time as a result of interpersonal communication. Communication can be verbal or nonverbal, but without some type of communication, there is no relationship.

## RELATIONSHIP: THE CIRCUIT FOR COMMUNICATION

A relationship is a "connection between people in which the participants have some degree of influence on each other's thoughts, feelings, and even actions" (VandenBos, 2009, p. 351). The key concept is *influential connection*. For purposes of illustration, the function of a relationship (or connection) between a provider and an older adult can be compared to an electric circuit.

The basic purpose of an electric circuit is to transport electricity—to make possible the flow of electricity between point A and point B. If a circuit exists, electricity can flow. If no circuit exists, no flow is possible. In a similar fashion, the purpose of a relationship is to transport interpersonal communication—to make possible the flow of communication between person A and person B. If a relationship exists, communication can flow. If no relationship exists, no flow of interpersonal communication is possible.

If problems exist within an electrical circuit, the flow of electricity can be hindered, degraded, or interrupted. Similarly, if problems exist within a relationship, the flow of communication can be impeded or interrupted. Cultivation and maintenance of a respectful, authentic, provider–older adult relationship is crucial to the success of a person-centered philosophy of communication and service delivery.

## PROFESSIONAL RELATIONSHIPS AND PERSON-CENTERED PHILOSOPHY

Person-centered service is a philosophy that views an older adult as a person first and as a patient, client, customer, or facility resident second. As a practical philosophy, it places the older person at the heart of any decision that would impact him or her. Inviting authentic collaboration, it views the older adult as an active partner in the process of satisfying his or her needs.

*Person-centered care is not about simply giving patients whatever they want, nor about merely providing information. It is about considering patients' preferences, values, family situations, social circumstances and lifestyles; seeing people as individuals and then working together to develop appropriate solutions (de Silva, 2014, p. 6).*

The person-centered approach—emphasizing compassion, dignity, and empathy—is increasingly acknowledged as one of the best evidence-based approaches to providing care and service (Edvardsson, Fetherstonhaugh, Nay, & Gibson, 2010). It is frequently employed as a key benchmark for measuring healthcare system delivery improvement (de Silva, 2014). The Accreditation Council on Graduate Medical Education (ACGME) and the American Board of Medical Specialties (ABMS) have identified communication skill as a core competency (National Institute on Aging, 2011).

## DEFINITIONS AND DESCRIPTIONS OF PERSON-CENTERED CARE

The United States Institute of Medicine developed a definition of quality in healthcare that enjoys widespread global acceptance. This description identifies compassionate, respectful, person-centered care as one of the necessary features required for delivery of high-quality care.

A project was discussed by de Silva (2014) that summarized results from over 23,000 separate studies that focused on various aspects of person-centered care. Several common themes were identified: compassion, dignity, patient involvement, person-centered communication, respect, shared decision-making, and provider support of patient self-empowerment and self-management.

Although no universally accepted definitions of person-centered care yet exist, there are widely agreed upon objectives. These include the following:

- Getting to know the older adult as a person—recognizing his or her individuality and uniqueness.
- Recognizing the older adult's autonomy—sharing power and responsibility for decision making.
- Having supportive staff—well trained in relationship-building and communication skills—who strive to put the older adult at the center of their focus.
- Establishing a collaborative and respectful partnership between service provider and older adult—a mutual effort in which the service provider respects the contribution the older adult can make to the satisfaction of need or resolution of his or her concern, combined with the older adult's respect of the provider for the contribution he or she can make toward the resolution of concerns.

For the provider, developing a respectful, working relationship with the older adult is critical to the rendering of satisfactory service. As Hart (2010) reminds, "It is the provider's responsibility to facilitate the establishment of a quality relationship with the client" (p. 170).

## PERSON CENTERED OR PROVIDER CENTERED?

Person-centered communication makes the older adult the central focus of the provider's attention. It places a high value on what the older adult communicates. This is in contrast to a provider-centered approach where most of the attentional and information value is placed on the provider. Using a person-centered approach requires striking a respectful balance between the autonomy of the older adult and the authority of the provider to achieve a mutually satisfactory service outcome (Phelps & Hassed, 2012).

To respect the autonomy of the older adult, it is not necessary (or desirable) for the provider to abdicate professional responsibility. Central to the person-centered approach is an ongoing collaboration between the provider and older adult where each uses his or her respective expertise to inform and guide the process. Example: A pharmacist brings pharmaceutical expertise to the interaction, and the older adult customer brings expertise regarding his or her background: known allergies; current symptoms, concerns, or problems; and subjective and objective experience with various medications.

## PERSON-CENTERED, RELATIONSHIP-BASED SERVICE DELIVERY

Person-centered service delivery places the needs of the older adult ahead of any other agenda. The focus is first and foremost on the *person*, then on his or her *concerns*, and finally on formulating a mutually agreed upon plan of intervention or action.

A person-centered approach involves "treating people as individuals; looking at the world from the perspective of the older person; involving the older person in decision-making; and challenging stereotypes about aging" (Waring, 2012, p. 24). In a person-centered relationship there is no "one size fits all."

Providers frequently voice the concern that adopting a patient-centered, individualized approach will require too much additional time—a commodity often in short supply. Evidently, this concern is mostly unfounded. Phelps & Hassed (2012) report that numerous studies have demonstrated a negligible increase in the length of interactions by those using this approach.

## THE ROLE OF RAPPORT IN ESTABLISHING A PERSON-CENTERED RELATIONSHIP

The contextual foundation for person-centered communication is a person-centered relationship—a concept grounded in the work of American psychologist Carl Rogers. Relationships develop through a felt sense of connection. Connection is largely developed through the process of cultivating rapport.

Rapport is defined as, "a warm, relaxed relationship of mutual understanding, acceptance, and sympathetic compatibility between or among individuals" (VandenBos, 2009, p. 342). Underscoring the importance of establishing a state of rapport, a popular saying declares, "With rapport nearly anything is possible. Without rapport almost nothing is possible."

## THE NATURE OF RAPPORT

Rapport is one of the key ingredients of a satisfying relationship (Cooper, 2008). When people are in a state of rapport, each party in the conversation is listening to the other, and each knows he or she is being listened to by the other (Ready & Burton, 2004).

Individuals in a state of rapport often feel more connected—as if they are on the same "wavelength." They sense a sharing of common ground (Brooks, 1991). This frequently results in each person perceiving the other as being more likeable—an interesting phenomenon with practical applications in light of evidence that suggests people tend to *like* people who like them and like people who are *like* them (Cialdini, 2009).

## ESTABLISHING RAPPORT IN AN UNEQUAL RELATIONSHIP

When a provider and older adult interact, the professional is often perceived as the one having the most control, knowledge, and/or skill. Based on this imbalance of control or power, the relationship is often experienced as hierarchical and unequal. Tamparo and Lindh (2008) insist that even the widely used terms *patient* or *client* imply a hierarchical relationship. This perceived inequality can function as a barrier to establishing or deepening rapport and as a stumbling block on the path to building a well-functioning professional relationship.

The older adult who presents with a need or who is seeking help is routinely judged as being less empowered than the professional who can address the need or provide the sought-after help. Providers who adopt a person-centered approach—and who seek to develop the necessary rapport to build a relationship—need to remain sensitive and aware of this perceived power differential and do everything reasonably possible to help the older adult feel more empowered.

## THEORIES OF AGING AND PERSON-CENTERED COMMUNICATION

A theory is "a principle or body of interrelated principles that purport to explain or predict a number of interrelated phenomena" (VandenBos, 2009, p. 426). Theories provide a lens through which a topic may be viewed.

There are numerous psychosocial theories of aging. The select theories mentioned in this chapter were chosen to serve as examples illustrating how the actions and attitudes of an older adult can be interpreted differently depending on the particular theory embraced by the provider. In this context, a theory of aging functions much like the concept of *worldview* explored in Chapter 2.

It is not the purpose or focus of this book to summarize the major theories of aging. Nevertheless, it is important to explicitly identify the major theoretical underpinnings of this work. The overall conceptual framework for this book is rooted in a bio–psycho–social perspective of aging.

The argument for a person-centered approach to communication was heavily influenced by the seminal work of Carl Rogers.

## THE INFLUENCE OF AGING THEORIES IN ESTABLISHING RAPPORT

An older adult may hold differing views and face different developmental life tasks (agendas) from members of other age groups.

When a provider is aware of and understands some of these basic differences, the process of establishing rapport can be hastened. If a provider lacks awareness and understanding of these differences, the process of establishing rapport can be impeded.

Erik Erikson (1902–1994) was a psychologist who explored these differing, age-related developmental agendas (Erikson, 1959). His eight-stage theory of aging is currently a widely used model.

## ERIK ERIKSON'S EIGHT-STAGE THEORY OF PSYCHOSOCIAL DEVELOPMENT

According to Erikson's theory, individuals pass through eight major life stages on their psychosocial journey from infancy to death (Harwood, 2007). Each of these stages involves confrontation with two conflicting developmental tasks. Erikson referred to a conflicting task as a crisis—a psychological conundrum that must be resolved in order for the individual to successfully move forward to the next stage of personal development.

The crisis faced at the eighth stage by the adult aged 65 and older was coined *Ego Integrity* versus *Despair*. Erikson believed that the older adult reflects back over his or her life and, as a result, feels either mostly satisfied or mostly dissatisfied. If the older adult judges life to have been meaningful, productive, and successful, a deep satisfaction is experienced, and the process of ego integrity continues. If, on the other hand, the older adult judges his or her life to have been unproductive, unsuccessful, and lacking in meaning, a deep dissatisfaction or despair ensues and the process of ego integrity is impeded.

There are those who believe Erikson's theory may now be somewhat outdated. They argue that his work failed to recognize the possibility for continued developmental challenges late into old age, and his final stage of development puts too much emphasis on achieving a final resolution and closure rather than engaging in a continued challenge (Harwood, 2007, p. 16).

The author—during his work as a medical social worker serving hospice patients with a terminal diagnosis—often observed older adults providing counsel to loved ones. Discussion of living an authentic life of purpose was a frequent theme. The importance of physical health, relationships, and pursuing personally meaningful activity was often stressed. The message frequently communicated by a patient near death to a loved one could be summed up by this quote supposedly made by Elvis Presley that what really matters is having "someone to love, something to do, and something to look forward to."

---

### Exercise: Reflect Once More on the Case Example of the Pharmacy Technician and the Mother-in-Law Presented in Chapter 2

1. Do you think if the provider (the pharmacy tech) had been aware of Erikson's theory about the psychosocial challenges faced by the older adult (the mother-in-law) that he may have displayed more patience? Why or why not?

2. Pretend that the mother-in-law—as she was standing at the counter nervously rummaging through her purse—had in the previous minutes, while waiting in line, been wondering if her life still mattered. How might the pharmacy tech's treatment of her influence the answer to her question?

3. Imagine you are the pharmacy tech. Before waiting on each new customer, you take a moment to mentally remind yourself, "The next person who steps up to the counter is wondering if his or her life really matters." How might that realization affect the quality of customer service? Now, acknowledge the fact that you don't know what the next customer is thinking and that how you treat him or her might have unforeseen repercussions.

The intention of this exercise is to help illustrate and emphasize how theory can influence behavior—of how the actions and attitudes of an older adult can be interpreted differently depending on the particular theory (or worldview) embraced by the provider.

## ADDITIONAL METHODS FOR CULTIVATING RAPPORT

Rapport can be cultivated in a number of ways—a friendly smile, body turned toward the older adult, or gentle eye contact. Rapport may also begin to develop and deepen when a provider and older adult discover they share the following:

- Mutual friends or acquaintances.
- Similar backgrounds, places lived, schools attended, or places visited.
- Similar interests in certain types of pets.
- Similar hobbies, sports, or recreational interests.
- Membership in the same social, charitable, military, political, or religious organizations.
- Similar medical or other concerns.

Rapport may also be enhanced when individuals discover they have a common skill set, share similar values and beliefs, or shared enthusiasm for something (Ready & Burton, 2004).

## DEEPENING RAPPORT

There are many ways to deepen rapport. Probably the most common way simply involves the passage of time combined with numerous encounters and pleasant interactions. This is an example of a powerful learning principle in action—spaced repetition with intermittent reinforcement over time. In other words, the provider and older adult have a number of interactions over a period of weeks or months (spaced repetition) that, for the most part, result in mutually satisfying interactions (intermittent reinforcement). This particular pattern of "exposure" (contact) to a "situation" (such as a visit to physician) and reward often results in strong positive behavioral conditioning (a good feeling by the person) and offers one explanation for how friendships develop (the patient feels good about returning to the doctor). The identification of the constructive effect of spaced repetition and intermittent positive reinforcement on the learning process is attributed to an observation made by Hermann Ebbinghaus in the 1800s (Ebbinghaus, 1913).

To deepen rapport, the provider can express a genuine interest in learning more about the older adult—about what is important to him or her. The emphasis is upon the provider making a greater effort to better understand the older adult, not the older adult understanding the provider.

Another suggestion is to listen carefully to the manner of speaking used by the older adult and, if and when appropriate, to *slightly* reflect some of the noted characteristics. This extremely subtle process of imitating is often referred to as *mirroring*.

## RAPPORT AND MIRRORING

During interactions with an older adult, it is important for the provider to mindfully pay attention to the content of what is being communicated. In terms of rapport, it is also helpful to give some attention to the older adult's process of communicating—to be aware of some of the audio characteristics of the individual's voice. Examples of characteristics to listen for include the following:

• Tempo of speech: How fast does the individual tend to speak? Does his or her overall rate of speech seem to be slow or fast?

• Volume of speech: How loudly does the person tend to speak? Is his or her voice softer or louder?

• Tonality: What is the tonal quality of the person's voice? Does the older adult tend to speak using a monotone or singsong voice?

After listening carefully to the voice of the older adult and identifying some of his or her speaking characteristics, the provider may choose to make subtle adjustments to the tempo, volume, and tonality of some of his or her own speech to more closely match that of the older adult. The emphasis is on the word *some*. It is not mocking.

This is a subtle mirroring process often employed by psychologists, counselors, and by many other human services professionals. It is one practical application of the evidence-based finding that people tend to like people who like them and who are like them (Cialdini, 2009). Similarity matters.

It is strongly recommended that the provider interested in utilizing the technique of mirroring when engaged in professional interaction with older adults first practice this technique with family, friends, and/or colleagues. This is to help ensure that this subtle level of mirroring remains outside the conscious awareness of the person being mirrored. Information about the technique of mirroring can be researched in the body of literature on *neuro-linguistic programming*.

In addition to mirroring some of the vocal characteristics of the older adult, it might also prove helpful to notice the individual's preferences for *how* information is processed. Does he or she seem to prefer "the big picture" or a lot of detail? Once the provider has a sense of the older adult's preference, he or she could try offering information in the "portion size" they seem to prefer. This could be considered another form of mirroring.

The provider could also observe the older adult's overall posture, stance, and other nonverbal features of the communication process. Within the limits of professionalism and appropriateness, the provider could try adopting a similar stance, posture, and the occasional use of other nonverbal language such as gestures. Again, this is a subtle and somewhat advanced process, and it should be used sparingly, done only after additional study and practice or not at all.

Some additional ways to cultivate rapport include demonstrating respect for the older adult's sense of time, space, and money (Ready & Burton, 2004). There should be no obvious mimicry. This is not a game. A little bit of nonverbal mirroring goes a long way! The goal is to deepen rapport by subtly demonstrating similarity—people tend to like people who are like them.

Reflect for a moment on the story of the pharmacy technician and the mother-in-law from Chapter 2. Imagine how differently this interaction might have unfolded if the customer had simply felt seen, heard, and understood.

---

### Exercise: Compare and Contrast the Experience of Rapport with the Experience of Lack of Rapport

1. Bring to mind a personal professional relationship where you experienced the state of rapport. Review the explanation for how rapport evolves, and then reflect on how rapport was established in the relationship you selected. What was said or done (or not said and done) that resulted in the development of rapport?

2. Recall an interaction with a professional where no rapport was experienced. Identify what was said or done (or not said and done) that interfered with the cultivation of rapport. What created the lack of rapport?

3. Compare and contrast the differences between these two professional relationships. What do you notice?

## DON'T CALL ME HONEY!

What is in a name? Rapport! Unless an older adult requests to be called by something other than his or her given name, doing so could impede the evolving process of establishing rapport. In most cases, referring to an older adult as "honey" or "sweetie" (instead of using their name) during an interaction is inappropriate. More than inappropriate, it is often considered a display of ageism. It can be viewed as a form of *elderspeak*.

Elderspeak refers to the tendency of some individuals to inappropriately adjust their speech patterns when communicating with older adults. Often resembling "baby talk," it includes speaking more slowly, shortening sentences, or using limited or less complex vocabulary (VandenBos, 2009). Elderspeak is a rampant problem within the network of providers serving the needs of older adults.

It is important to find out how the older adult wants to be addressed. This is best done during the first meeting if possible. The simplest way to discover the older adult's preferences is to ask. Some individuals prefer a more formal approach—to be addressed by their surname and/or professional title (Mr, Mrs, or Dr). Others may feel more comfortable on a first name basis or have no preference.

The cliché, "You never get a second chance to make a good first impression," underscores the importance of getting it correct the first time. The topics of ageism, ageist attitudes, and the widespread problem of provider usage of elderspeak will be discussed in detail in a later chapter.

## THE ROLE OF DEEP LISTENING IN RAPPORT BUILDING

The skill of deep listening is critical to the person-centered approach to communication and service delivery. *Deep listening* is defined as being able to pay attention to both the content and the process of what an individual is communicating. In the context of cultivating rapport, deep listening means paying full attention to *what* the older adult is communicating (the message) and also attending to the aspects of *how* the message is being communicated (the process).

When a provider combines deep listening, keen observation, and appropriate use of questions with the sharing of information relevant to the older adult's concerns, this can result in an increase in rapport—the foundation and glue of a provider–older adult relationship. It should also foster cultivation of a more satisfying interpersonal communication experience—an experience where the older adult feels seen, heard, and understood. This is where the concept of *mindfulness* is important.

## PERSON-CENTERED MINDFULNESS

In the process of establishing rapport, building a mutually satisfying professional relationship, and engaging in person-centered communication, paying attention to the older adult when he or she is speaking is critically important. Individuals engaged in conversation can nearly always sense if the listener is truly paying attention. When a person believes he or she is being mindfully listened to, rapport is enhanced.

Mindfulness is "living in the *what-is* as opposed to the *what-if*" (Altman, 2014, p. 3). Stewart (2004) describes mindfulness as being in the present moment with bare attention. Bare attention can be understood as the full and undistorted awareness of moment-by-moment experience (Silananda, 1990).

Govinda (1975) describes mindfulness as the ability to experience the present moment without the distortion caused by memory or imagination. Mindfulness is experiencing the unfolding moment with no effort to analyze, describe, compare, categorize, or interpret it. The provider who is listening mindfully to an older adult client or customer is paying attention to what is being said and how it is being said. He or she is actively engaged in the act of listening in the present moment—something the older adult can usually sense.

Dixit (2008) points out the obvious—life unfolds only in the present moment. At times—due to worry about the imagined future or rumination over the remembered past—the present moment can slip by unnoticed.

Mindfulness is moment-to-moment awareness of life as it is. It is an open, receptive, and non-judging awareness (Kornfield, 1993).

The quality of non-judging awareness is in contrast to the practice of mental labeling, judging, and interpreting of experience. For example, in Chapter 2, when the pharmacy technician was trying to help the mother-in-law, a more mindful approach might have led to a more desirable outcome. Had he been more mindful, the pharmacy technician might have ignored thoughts such as "Boy, this old woman is sure slow; if she doesn't speed things up, my other customers are really going to get mad!" Instead, he might have simply focused on what was needed to provide an excellent customer experience.

A mindful approach is focused solely on "what is" not on how things "should be." The non-mindful approach is influenced by the mental overlay of beliefs and expectations about what "ought" to be or how things "should" proceed. This overlay functions as a barrier to effectively dealing with the way things "are" and can trigger mental processes that label (e.g., "This old woman"), interpret, and judge ("If she doesn't speed things up, my other customers are really going to get mad"). These are ageist views that can negatively impact the quality-of-service delivery.

Much scientific research has been conducted measuring the efficacy of mindfulness-based interventions. Numerous meta-analyses and systematic reviews support the use of mindfulness for a variety of applications (Goldberg, Del Re, Hoyt, & Davis, 2014). A comprehensive meta-analysis of 209 studies involving a total of over 12,000 participants concluded that Mindfulness-Based Therapy is an effective treatment for a variety of psychological problems, and it is especially effective for reducing anxiety, depression, and stress (Khoury et al., 2013). Links to reviews that examine some of the evidence can be accessed at Mindfulness Research Center Web site http://www.mindfulexperience.org/evidence-base.php.

The topic of mindfulness has a large and growing body of literature. For providers interested in empirical measures of mindfulness, a list of many instruments are available at the Web site for the Mindfulness Resource Guide http://www.mindfulexperience.org/measurement.php.

## MULTITASKING VERSUS MINDFULNESS

Standing in sharp contrast to the practice of mindfulness is the so-called skill of *multitasking*. Multitasking refers to an individual's supposed ability to engage in two or more conscious tasks concurrently. Empirically based doubt has been cast on the concept of conscious multitasking.

Moran (2007) reported on research supported by funding from the National Institute of Mental Health. In this study, neuroscientists from Vanderbilt University were able to identify the areas of the brain that interfere with being able to consciously do two or more things at once. Using functional magnetic resonance imaging, they examined neural activity over time. Their research provides neurological evidence that suggests the brain cannot effectively engage in more than one conscious activity at a time.

Crenshaw (2008) explained that what is commonly referred to as multitasking is more accurately explained as a process of rapid toggling back and forth between different tasks. This toggling process is known as *switch tasking*. It is commonly believed that multitasking can help save time, but the act of switching actually results in a loss of time and attention. When a provider toggles back and forth between activities, he or she often has to quickly review what has already been completed before work can resume. This review requires time. The more complicated the task, the more time is lost from switching or multitasking.

Moran (2007) discussed research that also suggests that attempts to multitask can trigger the stress response and increase the probability of making errors. Apparently, the stress response is triggered by the rapid and repeated toggling back and forth between two or more tasks—an important concept that will be discussed later in this book.

---

### Author's Personal Observation Serving as a Home Health and Hospice Medical Social Worker

Many patients expressed their dislike of providers who would spend more time looking at their laptop, computer, or tablet than at them. This is a common practice in some hospitals, clinics, and other facilities. Examples include providers who document services or enter chart notes on a laptop computer or tablet during the appointment instead of after. Patients often reported feeling distanced and disrespected due to the attention the provider was giving to the devices instead of to them.

They reported that providers often had a tendency to talk "at them" rather than "with them." Providers would ask questions and type in the patient's response with very little eye contact. Patient's views were shared with staff, and the staff reply was often the same, "I know patients don't like it when we complete our patient visit notes during the visit instead of after, but that's the way we've been instructed to do it. It supposedly saves time."

**Author's professional opinion:** Provider use of laptops, tablets, and smart cell phones in front of an older adult is often viewed as rude and disrespectful. It is counterproductive to the process of developing rapport and to the practice of person-centered communication and service delivery. Making small changes to the interaction with the older adult can make a big difference. As an example, the provider could first make eye contact with the older adult, smile, and ask an engaging open-ended question. When documentation is required, the provider could mention, giving undivided attention, the importance of accurate chart notes to quality care, that it will only take a couple of minutes, and when finished he or she will again have the provider's full attention.

---

## SERVICE IN THE DIGITAL AGE

New technologies are on the horizon. Extraordinary developments in the use of artificial intelligence and robotics, genomics and biotechnology, nanotechnology, virtual exam and treatment rooms, sophisticated sensors, home diagnostics and personal monitoring systems are laying the foundation for an era of highly personalized, home-based services, especially in the fields of education and health care (Huston, 2013).

These breakthrough developments could lead to an era of home-based service delivery that is personal, participatory, predictive, and preventative.

A possible portend of things to come, in Japan, robots are already beginning to be used to care for the elderly (Huston, 2013).

The argument made in this book is that even in the most hi-tech environment of the future, it will still be important to do the following:

- Get to know the older adult as a person—recognizing his or individuality and uniqueness.
- Recognize the older adult's autonomy—sharing power and responsibility for decision making.
- Have supportive staff that are well trained in relationship building and communication skills—who strive to put the older adult at the center of their focus.
- Establish a collaborative and respectful partnership between service provider and older adult—a mutual effort in which the service provider respects the contribution the older adult can make to the satisfaction of need or resolution of his or her concern, combined with the older adult's respect of the provider for the contribution he or she can make toward the resolution of their concerns.

## CONCLUSION

Whether the provider–older adult interaction takes place physically face-to-face or digitally face-to-face, cultivating a rapport-based professional relationship in which respectful, person-centered communication can occur will likely remain the gold standard of quality service. The next chapter focuses on the "nuts-and-bolts" of interpersonal communication.

## LIST OF MAIN POINTS FOR PREVIEW AND REVIEW

- The compassionate, collaborative, empathetic, person-centered approach is acknowledged as one of the best evidence-based approaches to providing service.
- Person-centered service views an older adult as a person first and as a patient, client, customer, or facility resident second. It places the older person at the heart of decisions that would impact him or her.
- Communication occurs within a relationship.
- Establishing a rapport-based relationship is the probably the provider's most important task.
- Relationships develop from communication and a felt sense of connection.
- Connection is developed from rapport and through deep listening.

- Rapport is a warm, relaxed relationship of mutual understanding, acceptance, and sympathetic compatibility between individuals.
- *Deep listening* is being able to pay attention to both the content and the process of what an individual is communicating.
- Cultivation and maintenance of a respectful provider–older adult relationship is crucial to the success of person-centered, interpersonal communication and service delivery.

## Provider Self-Test and/or Discussion Suggestions for Instructors

**Discuss:** The importance and benefits of a rapport-based professional relationship with an older adult.

**Explain:** How professional relationships develop. Be certain to address the role of rapport, connection, and communication.

**Discuss:** The philosophy of person-centered care. Identify key characteristics. Differentiate person centered from provider centered, giving examples of each.

**List:** Several ways that rapport may be developed and deepened.

**Explain:** The process of *mirroring*, what it is used for, and how it is done.

**Discuss:** The importance of calling an individual by his or her name. Integrate the concept of *elderspeak* into your discussion.

**Define:** The concepts of *deep listening, multitasking,* and *mindfulness.* Talk about their role in the process of cultivating rapport.

## WEB RESOURCES

### Person-Centered Care
Institute for Person-Centered Care
  http://ubipcc.com/
The Association for the Development of the Person-Centered Approach
  http://www.adpca.org/

### Mindfulness Research
  http://www.mindfulexperience.org/

## REFERENCES

Altman, D. (2014). *The mindfulness toolbox: 50 practical tips, tools, and handouts for anxiety, depression, and pain.* Eau Claire, WI: PESI Publishing.
Brooks, M. (1991). *The power of business rapport.* New York: HaperCollins Publishers.
Cialdini, R. B. (2009). *Influence: Science and practice.* New York: Pearson Education, Inc.

Cooper, L. (2008). *Business NLP for dummies.* West Sussex, England: John Wiley & Sons, Ltd.

Crenshaw, D. (2008). *The myth of multitasking.* San Francisco: Jossey-Bass.

Dixit, J. (2008). The art of now. *Psychology Today,* 64–69.

Ebbinghaus, H. (1913). *Memory. A contribution to experimental psychology.* New York: Columbia University (Reprinted Bristol: Thoemmes Press, 1999).

Edvardsson, D., Fetherstonhaugh, D., Nay, R., & Gibson, S. (2010). Development and initial testing of the Person-centered Care Assessment Tool (P-CAT). *International Psychogeriatrics, 22*(1), 101–108.

Erikson, E. H. (1959). *Identity and the life cycle.* New York: International Universities Press.

Hart, V. A. (2010). *Patient-provider communications: Caring to listen.* Sudbury, MA: Jones and Bartlett Publishers.

Harwood, J. (2007). *Understanding communication and aging.* Thousand Oaks, CA: Sage Publications.

Huston, C. (2013). The impact of emerging technology on nursing care: warp speed ahead. *OJIN: The Online Journal of Issues in Nursing, 18*(2). http://dx.doi.org/10.3912/OJIN.Vol18No02Man01.

Goldberg, S. B., Del Re, A. C., Hoyt, W. T., & Davis, J. M. (2014). The secret ingredient in mindfulness interventions? A case for practice quality over quantity. *Journal of Counseling Psychology, 61*(3), 491–497.

Govinda, A. (1975). *Foundations of Tibetan mysticism.* New York: Weiser.

Khoury, B., Lecomte, T., Fortin, G., Masse, M., Therien, P., Bouchard, V., et al. (2013). Mindfulness-based therapy: a comprehensive meta-analysis. *Clinical Psychology Review, 33*(6), 763–771.

Kornfield, J. (1993). *A path with a heart: A guide through the perils and promises of spiritual life.* New York: Bantam.

Moran, M. (2007). *Researchers find neural 'bottleneck' thwarts multitasking.* http://www.vanderbilt.edu/register/articles?id=31525.

National Institute on Aging. (2011). *Talking with your older patient: A clinician's handbook* Kindle edition.

Phelps, K., & Hassed, C. (2012). *Communication with patients.* Kindle edition. Chatswood, NSW: Elsevier, Australia.

Ready, R., & Burton, K. (2004). *Neuro-linguistic programming for dummies.* West Sussex, England: John Wiley & Sons, Ltd.

Silananda, U. (1990). *The four foundations of mindfulness.* Boston, MA: Wisdom Publications.

de Silva, D. (2014). *Helping measure person-centered care: A review of evidence about commonly used approaches and tools used to help measure person-centered care.* London, UK: The Health Foundation. www.health.org.uk. 1–76.

Stewart, T. (2004). Acceptance through mindfulness. *Behavior Modification, 28*(6), 783–811.

Tamparo, C. D., & Lindh, W. Q. (2008). *Therapeutic communications for healthcare.* Clifton Park, New York: Thompson Delmar Learning.

VandenBos, G. R. (Ed.). (2009). *APA college dictionary of psychology.* Washington, DC: American Psychological Association.

Waring, A. (2012). *The heart of care.* London, England: Souvenir Press.

CHAPTER 4

# Nuts and Bolts of Interpersonal Communication: The Clinical Face of Service

*The art of conversation lies in listening.*

*Malcolm Forbes*

**Core Question:** What are the main characteristics of effective, respectful, person-centered communication?

**Keywords:** Communication; Deep listening; Elderspeak; Message fidelity; Mindfulness; Mirroring; Multitasking; Nonverbal communication; Paraphrasing; Rapport.

## INTRODUCTION

This chapter provides the "nuts and bolts" of the person-centered approach to communication. It discusses a simple model of interaction the provider can use to frame his or her interactions with older adults.

### PROVIDER–OLDER ADULT INTERPERSONAL COMMUNICATION

Numerically speaking, the most widely used clinical skills within the healthcare system are communication skills (Bras, Dordevic, & Janjanin, 2013). Qualitatively speaking, increasing numbers of older adults feel dissatisfied with the caliber of the communication skills demonstrated by their providers (Moses, 2005). This book was written to assist providers, administrators, and educators who want to improve these clinical skills or assist others to do so.

Chapter 1 explained that this dissatisfaction can be traced to the collective experiences of older adults interacting with providers whose schedules seem to leave only enough time for rushed, overly technical, disrespectful, and occasionally ageist conversations. These experiences have left many older adults feeling angry, frustrated, and disempowered. As an antidote to this growing

*Person-Centered Communication with Older Adults*
http://dx.doi.org/10.1016/B978-0-12-420132-3.00004-0
55

concern, Chapter 1 recommended providers adopt a respect-based, person-centered, plain-language approach to communicating with older adults.

Methods that providers can use to help acquire or improve person-centered communication skills were described in Chapter 2. This included suggestions for how to recognize and modify potentially limiting personal views, methods for examining individual motivations for wanting to learn, ways to identify current communication strengths, and strategies for developing a targeted professional improvement plan. Many of these methods can be adapted to assist with implementation of organizational change.

Chapter 3 focused on how to establish a rapport-based professional relationship. The practitioner's best chance for developing rapport comes from well-developed communication skills (Meldrum, 2005).

A key to the communicating process, the provider–older adult relationship was characterized, not only as the foundation for person-centered service delivery, but as the vehicle for effective and meaningful interaction.

This chapter focuses on the "nut and bolts" of what transpires within that relationship—interpersonal communication. Spitzberg and Cupach (1984) identified three basic requirements for providers wanting to communicate competently: desire, knowledge, and skill.

1. Desire: The provider must want to communicate effectively and appropriately with older adults.
2. Knowledge: The provider needs to understand what information and skills are required to communicate effectively and appropriately.
3. Skill: The provider must possess the skill sets typically associated with effective, competent communication.

## THE TWO FACES OF SERVICE: TECHNICAL AND CLINICAL

Under the umbrella known as the network of aging-services providers, are professionals and members as numerous and diverse as the elderly adults they serve. These providers have at least two responsibilities in common:

1. They all serve older adults.
2. The services rendered are dual in nature—they have a technical face and a clinical face.

The technical face of service refers to all the specialized skills, instruments, and equipment involved in providing diagnoses, treatments, and interventions. Technical service is most recognizable in the healthcare sector. The clinical face of service refers to all the specialized skills involved in human relations—cultivating rapport, developing a professional relationship—all the nuts and bolts of a person-centered communication approach designed to help older adults address their concerns.

Unfortunately, although the clinical needs of older adults are often as important as the technical needs, it is the clinical needs that frequently receive far too little attention. This chapter focuses on how to improve the clinical face of service delivery—professional provider communication.

## PROFESSIONAL PROVIDER COMMUNICATION VERSUS SOCIAL COMMUNICATION

Professional provider communication differs from nonprofessional social communication. Social communication occurs between family, friends, and other acquaintances. Within the domain of the aging services network, professional communication takes place between an older adult who has a specific need, concern, or problem and a skilled provider who can address that specific need, concern, or problem (Tamparo & Lindh, 2008).

Whether it involves a physician or phlebotomist; a pharmacist or medical aide; a nurse or physical therapist; an assisted living social director or driver for special needs transportation; provider communication requires specific, well-defined professional skills. Provider communication is purposeful and service-oriented and differentiates itself from nonprofessional, social communication.

## PURPOSEFUL COMMUNICATION: CONTENT AND RELATIONSHIP

Communication is defined as "a process by which information is exchanged between individuals through a common system of symbols, signs, or behavior" (Mish, 2009, p. 251). Interpersonal communication is the intentional exchange of information between a provider and one or more older adults. It is a skill that can be learned and developed. It is the means by which an individual expresses his or her thoughts, feelings, hopes, and aspirations within the context of a relationship.

This book presupposes that interpersonal communication is purposeful. It also assumes this purpose is dual in nature—providing topical information and relationship information. Paul Watzlawick (1967) in his classic treatise on interpersonal communication *The Pragmatics of Human Communication* argued that communication is always two-fold—always about the message and the relationship.

Purposeful communication can be used constructively and destructively. It can help and harm. On the more constructive and helpful side, providers commonly use communication for the following:
• asking questions, discovering information;
• expressing caring, compassion, curiosity, and respect;
• sharing information, concerns, opinions, experiences, and examples;
• describing, explaining, educating, and instructing;
• coaching, encouraging, inspiring, and motivating; and
• convincing, influencing, persuading, and warning.

On the more destructive and harmful side, unfortunately, some providers occasionally use communication for these purposes:
• belittling, blaming, and bullying;
• criticizing and judging;
• commanding, directing, and over-controlling;
• lying, manipulating;
• demonstrating non-caring, cruelty, and disrespect; and
• spreading gossip, hurtful rumors, discrimination, prejudice and hate.

Whether verbal, nonverbal, or text-based—purposeful, respectful, person-centered, service-oriented communication is the gold standard of provider communication.

## TYPES OF COMMUNICATION: VERBAL, NONVERBAL, AND TEXT-BASED

The focus of this chapter is on the purposeful, verbal, nonverbal, and text-based communication that occurs between providers and older adults. Text-based communication is used primarily when writing on paper or using a keyboard to enter information into a computer, tablet, or phone. Verbal communication is voice-based and includes the auditory qualities of vocal tonality and tempo. Nonverbal communication includes physical gestures, mannerisms, body posture, and spatial positioning. Of all the types of nonverbal messages, perhaps facial expressions are the most obvious nonverbal communicator.

For the provider, one of the most immediately useful applications of nonverbal communications is simply to notice whether the verbal and nonverbal communications appear to be congruent. Do they seem to match up and support one another or are they mismatched—seemingly conveying different or conflicting messages? Here is an exaggerated example to help make this distinction clear: A provider asks an older adult male how he feels. The older man verbally replies, "Fine," while nonverbally squirming in his chair, tears streaming down his reddened-face. The verbal message and the nonverbal communication do not appear to support each other. There is a mismatch. Continuing with the same example, if the older adult had answered, "Fine," while relaxing comfortably in his chair with a big authentic smile on his face, then it would appear his verbal and nonverbal communication are congruent and supportive of each other. When an apparent mismatch is observed, the provider's skillful use of appropriate comments and questions can often help clarify.

Providers are cautioned to bear in mind that nonverbal communication is easily and frequently misinterpreted. A full discussion of this topic is beyond the scope of this chapter. Those who desire additional information are encouraged to consult the large body of available literature.

## THE CYCLE OF COMMUNICATION

Provider communication is purposeful and occurs within the context of a professional interaction. The overall process of communicating is often described as a cycle.

Tamparo and Lindh (2008) describe this cycle as having four main components. These include the following:

1. The sender: This is the person speaking, gesturing, or writing—the source of the message.
2. The receiver: This is the person listening, viewing, or reading—the recipient of the message.
3. The message: This is the information being transmitted verbally, nonverbally, or via text.
4. The channel or mode of communication: This includes speaking, listening, writing, and gesturing.

## THE THREE COMPONENTS OF THE PROVIDER–OLDER ADULT INTERACTION

In this book, communication is envisioned as an interaction or encounter between a provider and an older adult. Although each encounter is unique, it can be understood as involving three basic steps that are repeated over and over again in every interaction that occurs in a professional relationship (Tamparo & Lindh, 2008).

As an example, an older adult comes in for an appointment.

1. During the first few moments of this interaction, the provider and the older adult begin to orient to each other. This is where relationship and rapport are initiated by such behaviors as eye contact, smiling, and saying "hello."

2. As the interaction continues, the provider and older adult use communication to identify the older adult's problem, concern, or need.

3. Once the problem, need, or concern has been identified, the provider attempts to address the older adult's concern.

This three-step model of interaction is a practical way of viewing the purpose of professional encounters. During all stages of the interaction—from beginning to end—what are referred to as the seven C's of communication play a significant role.

## THE SEVEN C'S OF EFFECTIVE, COMPETENT COMMUNICATION

There are several qualities associated with effective, person-centered interpersonal communication. In this chapter, these qualities are referred to as the seven C's of communication—so named because each word begins with the letter C. These qualities or traits are similar but not identical with those described by Tamparo and Lindh (2008) in their excellent book *Therapeutic Communication for the Health Professional*. The seven C's are as follows:

1. Caring: Effective communication is grounded in the provider's genuine caring or concern for the older adult. Listening is one way to demonstrate caring.

2. Compassionate: Effective, comforting communication expresses the compassion and empathy a provider feels for the older adult and his or her presenting need, problem, or concern.

3. Courteous: Effective communication demonstrates respect for the older adult. Listening is one way to demonstrate courteousness.

4. Clear: Effective communication is clear, unambiguous, void of unnecessary professional jargon, and easy to understand.

5. Concise: Effective communication is pithy, direct, and efficient.

6. Congruent: Effective communication is cohesive. Verbal and nonverbal communication deliver a message that support each other.

7. Complete: Effective communication has a beginning, a middle, and an end. It conveys a complete, cohesive story.

Within the context of the provider–older adult relationship, adhering to the above seven characteristics is one way a sender (the provider) can package his or her message to encourage *message fidelity*. Message fidelity is a term used to denote authentic information, with minimal distortion or compromise of meaning (Meldrum, 2005). Communication that supports message fidelity has a much better chance of reaching the receiver (the older adult) in the way the sender intended. This form of "packaging" also helps create and maintain rapport—so critical to the provider–older adult relationship.

## WAITING AND WAITING

Whether an older adult is sitting in the treatment room waiting for a physician, standing at the pharmacy counter waiting to talk with the pharmacist, or lying on the couch in an assisted-living apartment waiting for the night-shift aid to take a blood pressure reading, today's older adult seems to be forced to wait. Who can blame them for feeling disappointed, frustrated, hurt, or stressed when—after all that waiting—the provider finally arrives but then seems rushed, distant, and sometimes even disrespectful?

In contrast to the all too frequent provider–older adult interaction described above is the experience of 69-year-old Susan.

### Example of Susan

Susan reluctantly stopped by the medical clinic's lab to have some blood work completed that her physician had ordered. Susan had suffered many painful blood draws in the past and had a mild fear of needles.

After being greeted by a smiling receptionist, she sat down in the waiting room. A few minutes later, a door opened and a young woman who identified herself as a phlebotomist came out from the back of the lab. She escorted Susan to a straight-back chair where her blood would be drawn.

Evidently, the young woman sensed Susan was feeling nervous and politely asked if she would feel more comfortable sitting in the reclining chair that was located in a private area of the lab. Susan nodded her head affirmatively, and they walked to a curtained-off area where she took her seat in the recliner.

Speaking in a calm, relaxing voice, the phlebotomist initiated some small talk. Within a couple of minutes, Susan shared her fear of needles and, in turn, the phlebotomist shared her fear of dentists. She asked Susan if she'd prefer to have the blood taken from the left or right arm. Susan pointed to the left. The phlebotomist gently examined Susan's veins, applied some rubbing alcohol, and briefly explained the upcoming procedure—what she was going to do, how long it would take, and so forth—and then asked Susan if she was ready. Susan nodded, "Yes," and the phlebotomist proceeded with the blood draw.

After the procedure was completed and the phlebotomist was placing a small bandage on Susan's arm, she explained when the test results would be ready and asked if Susan had any final questions. She did not.

A few days later—during an interview for this book—when Susan was discussing her experience at the clinic lab, she added, "I could tell she cared about how nervous I felt. That by itself helped me to relax. She did not joke around in a loud voice like some of them do. She did not pretend that sticking a needle in my arm was not going to hurt. She took my nervousness seriously—treated me with respect. Her voice was very calming. That really helped! This was the easiest blood draw I've ever had!"

The blood draw was the technical side of the service, and the demeanor of the phlebotomist was the clinical side. As this example illustrates, when the technical aspect is rendered competently and the clinical side offered using a respectful, person-centered approach, the result can be a satisfied patient—a patient likely to share her favorable experience with family and friends.

In the preceding example, the phlebotomist demonstrated the principle of "first explain the procedure to the patient, then do it." Throughout her interaction with Susan, she wisely applied the seven *C*'s of communication.

### Exercise: Create a Professional Implementation Plan

Providers are encouraged to review the learning strategies explained in Chapter 2. Following the instructions provided, create a professional implementation plan focusing on developing competent understanding and application of the concepts and skill sets represented by the seven *C*'s. Most importantly (as soon as possible) begin to integrate and apply these concepts into the professional work setting. Intentionally and mindfully begin to integrate these person-centered qualities into the interpersonal communication process.

## THREE SPECIAL C'S

Because poor quality interpersonal communication can be a major source of stress and create significant problems for providers, older adults, and aging services–related organizations, Chapter 7 focuses on a special *C—calmness*. It includes detailed suggestions about how to develop a stress management plan of care—both for individual providers and employing organizations.

This $C$ is so important to the longterm health and success of the provider–older adult relationship (and the person-centered communication that takes place within it) that it is discussed separately from the seven $C$'s and has an entire chapter devoted to the topic.

Chapter 9 introduces the underappreciated but very important topic of neurocardiology and discusses the heart–brain partnership. How these two organs interact and the impact this interaction has on the communication process will be explored with emphasis on the concept of *coherence*—the next of the special $C$'s. Speculating on how energetic-based models of human connection might impact the provider–older adult relationship, Chapter 10 explores the physics of interpersonal communication and introduces the final $C$—*connection*.

## PERSON-CENTERED LISTENING

Listening is one of the major keys to the success of the person-centered approach to communication (Phelps & Hassed, 2012). Listening is a complex process combining hearing and understanding (Dreher, 2001). It is a search for meaning.

Probably the most common complaint expressed by older adults is that their provider does not listen to them. For example, some studies found that (on average) when healthcare professionals ask patients the opening question, nearly 75% interrupted the patient within 18 s (Phelps & Hassed, 2012). Frequently, after the interruption, the patient was never allowed to complete their story.

The person-centered provider listens intentionally and mindfully. With the ears, he or she listens for message content; with the heart, for feelings (see Chapter 9, *Neurocardiology and Communication*); and with the eyes, notices the accompanying nonverbal behavior.

The provider who is a mindful listener makes a sincere effort to keep his or her eyes on the speaker as much as possible—not a chart, laptop computer, smartphone, or tablet. A common complaint of many older adults sounds like this, "When I'm talking, they always seem to have their face buried in a chart or computer instead of paying attention to me. I hate that!"

Probably the most common (and the biggest) barrier to effective, person-centered listening is when the provider is thinking about something else while supposedly listening. This mind wandering can be rectified through practice of concentration and mindfulness.

Sometimes, while listening to an older adult speak, it can be challenging to refrain from mentally reviewing a recent conversation, from imagining an appointment scheduled later, or from indulging in thoughts and memories about personal affairs. Listening instead of speaking is often more difficult than it would seem. Providers are routinely trained to actively intervene with advice, suggestions, or prescriptions. But on occasion, none of these interventions are necessary. In these cases, the older adult simply needs someone to listen. Listening has its own place. Being listened to has its own value. The hardest part is doing it.

*Most people do not listen with the intent to understand; they listen with intent to reply.*
**Stephen Covey**

## SELF-ASSESSMENT: PROFESSIONAL LISTENING

- How would you rate your professional listening skills? How would the older adults you serve rate your listening skills?
- Mentally review a recent professional interaction where you felt disappointed in your listening skills. Do the same with a recent professional interaction where you felt proud of your listening skills. Compare the interaction you felt proud of with the disappointing interaction. How do they differ? If it was possible to go back in time and redo the disappointing interaction and transform it into an interaction that you could feel proud of, what would you change?
- What are one to two specific behaviors you could do (or not do) that you believe would improve your listening skills? As an option, you could skip ahead to Chapter 8 and use the mental imagery techniques explained in the section *Using Imagery and Daydreaming to Improve Communication* to imagine yourself as an excellent listener.

## ENCOURAGING ADDITIONAL DISCLOSURE AND ELABORATION

During the three-step model of interaction, the provider is using clinical skills—cultivating rapport, developing a professional relationship, all the nuts and bolts of a person-centered communication approach—to address the older adult's presenting need, concern, or problem. The provider relies on the skillful use of questions and mindful listening to assist in this endeavor.

As the interaction unfolds, it is common for the provider to encourage the older adult to elaborate upon and disclose additional information. There are many ways this can be accomplished respectfully. Four often used techniques are *observation, acknowledging feelings, clarifying*, and *paraphrasing*. Each provider will discover what feels best—and seems to work best—for him or her. Here are representative examples of each of these four "tools":

**Technique = Observation**

*Scenario*: During an interaction with the provider, an older adult male grimaces facially and groans. Using the technique of *observation*, the provider comments, "You seem uncomfortable."

**Technique = Acknowledging Feelings**

*Scenario*: During an interaction with the provider, an older adult woman (wringing her hands nervously) mentions having a problem with being able to afford her medications. Using the technique of *acknowledging feelings*, the provider comments, "Some of these medicines are pretty expensive. You seem worried about how you're going to pay for them."

**Technique = Clarifying**

*Scenario*: During an interaction with the provider, an older adult male mumbles something about his confusing new diet. Using the technique of *clarifying*, the provider comments, "I want to make sure I understand you. Are you telling me you feel confused about how to follow dietary instructions the nutritionist ordered for you?"

**Technique = Paraphrasing**

*Scenario*: During an interaction with the provider, an older adult female complains that she still hurts even after taking the pain pills. Using the technique of *paraphrasing*, the provider comments, "It sounds like you feel as if the pain meds are not helping like they should."

*Comment*: Many professionals are encouraged to use paraphrasing as a form of active listening. Paraphrasing means "listening to a speaker and then repeating what was said using different words" (Adams & Jones, 2011, p. 22).

The opinion offered in this book is that paraphrasing should be used sparingly—preferably only when a provider authentically feels it is necessary to confirm accurate understanding. However, paraphrasing in the form of a question might be appropriate when, for example, you see a grimace and ask, "Was there something you didn't understand or need me to go over more slowly?" When used for this purpose (as a tool for checking understanding) paraphrasing can also help build and maintain rapport. Appropriate paraphrasing demonstrates to the speaker that the provider is listening. It directs attention back to the speaker, demonstrates respect, conveys caring, and encourages the speaker to continue talking (Adams & Jones, 2011).

When used inappropriately—and especially when overused—paraphrasing comes off as parroting, which can be annoying to the patient. In this case, an older adult can feel as if a "technique" is being used on them, rather than feeling listened to and heard. If this occurs, rapport suffers. All four of these techniques—observation, acknowledging feelings, clarifying, and paraphrasing—when used authentically and sparingly in the service of improving communication, encourage the older adult to elaborate upon and disclose additional information and help the older adult to feel understood (Hart, 2010).

## THE THREE TYPES OF QUESTIONS IN THE PROVIDER–OLDER ADULT INTERACTION

Recall that earlier in this chapter, communication was envisioned as an interaction between a provider and an older adult that involved three basic steps—initial orientation to each other; identification of the older adult's problem, concern, or need; followed by the provider's attempt to address the older adult's concern. Throughout this interaction, the provider has three types of questions that can be asked to help build rapport and gather information relevant to the presenting issue. Knowing what type of question to ask—as well as when and how—requires much skill and experience.

It is helpful for the provider to consciously keep in mind the overall objective for asking questions, which is to help the older adult accurately express his or her need, concern, or problem and to discover information that might prove useful in helping to address the issue.

### Closed Questions

Closed questions are useful for quickly collecting information. Closed questions are questions that can be answered with a simple "Yes" or "No" or one word (Tamparo & Lindh, 2008). They often begin with words such as "do," "is," "are," "has," and "will." Some examples of closed questions include the following:

1. Do you have insurance?
2. Is your vision blurry?
3. Are you in any pain?
4. Has your hearing changed in the past six months?
5. Will you promise to take this medication every day?

Providers are cautioned that asking too many closed questions in a row can make many people feel as if they are being interrogated. This could result in the loss of rapport and negatively impact the professional relationship.

## Open-Ended Questions

Open-ended questions encourage the patient or client to provide more information than closed questions do. Open-ended questions cannot be answered with one word or "Yes" or "No." They often begin with words such as "how" or "what." Some examples of open-ended questions include these:
1. How did you initially respond to the doctor's diagnosis of your leg pain?
2. What seems to make your leg pain worse or better?

It is advisable to minimize use of questions that begin with the word "why." Questions that begin with "why" can trigger defensiveness (Tamparo & Lindh, 2008).

## Indirect Questions

Indirect questions are not really questions at all—they are statements that function like a question. They typically follow the use of a closed question or open-ended question and invite further disclosure and elaboration.

An indirect question makes a request for additional information without making the older adult feel as if they are being questioned (Tamparo & Lindh, 2008). They often begin with words or phrases such as "Tell me" or "I'm interested" or "I'd like." Some examples of indirect questions include the following:
1. Tell me more about your leg pain.
2. I'm interested in hearing about your experience with the physical therapist.
3. I'd like to hear what you think of your new diet.

The questions asked will determine the answers provided. The person-centered provider should be mindful of the information that he or she is seeking and then use the type of question that is best suited to elicit that information. In any event, the provider is encouraged to mix up the types of questions being asked. Not only does this variety help maintain a more relaxed flow of conversation, it also helps the older adult feel more comfortable, which can strengthen the professional relationship.

## SUGGESTIONS FOR EFFECTIVE, PERSON-CENTERED COMMUNICATION

The following suggestions can enhance the person-centered approach to communication. They can help providers cultivate rapport and support the professional relationship. When interacting with an older adult, do the following:
- Smile. Speak using plain, nontechnical, conversational language.
- Make sure your communication adheres to the seven C's.

- Speak more slowly if necessary. This is especially important with older adults who may have a hearing impairment or for those who evince a cognitive impairment.
- It can be useful to frame the upcoming conversation. Use the three-step approach: (1) describe what you will be talking about, (2) talk to the older adult about it, (3) and finish by summarizing what was discussed.
- Use the three types of questions—closed, open-ended, and indirect for gathering information.
- Limit the quantity of information shared. Check that the older adult understands what was communicated before giving additional information. Use the teach-back method. Example: Have the older adult describe what they understand. "Mr. Jones, when you get home, how will you explain these dietary changes to your wife?" This allows the provider to learn what the patient understands and to correct misunderstandings or provide missing information.
- When an older adult is speaking, use a listening posture. Lean slightly toward the older adult. Use head nods and the four techniques of observation, acknowledging feelings, clarifying, and paraphrasing to demonstrate listening and understanding. Remember to smile (Drench, Noonan, Sharby, & Ventura, 2012).

## BARRIERS TO EFFECTIVE, PERSON-CENTERED COMMUNICATION

Barriers to communication often interfere with rapport and can undermine the provider-older adult relationship. Some of the most common barriers to effective, person-centered communication are these:

- Talking about an older person in front of them or talking *for* them (unless requested to do so).
- Inappropriate use of professional jargon and unnecessary use of complex, technical explanations.
- Expressing ageism or ethnocentrism (see Chapter 5).
- Use of trite clichés, for example, "Don't worry. Everything will be all right." Clichés are often interpreted by the listener as a sign the provider does not understand or does not really care.
- Offering unwanted, unsolicited advice, lecturing, or moralizing: Providing advice often begins with words such as "If I were you."
- Belittling, shaming, and ridiculing: Provider use of belittling or shaming often begins with accusatory sounding phrases such as "Why would you

do such a thing?" Shaming or ridiculing might sound like this, "What possessed you to…" or "What were you thinking?"

- Contradicting, or criticizing: For example, an older woman was at her dentist having a tooth repaired. She was gripping the sides of the chair as if her life depended on it. Her face was red and eyes filled with tears. The dentist stopped the procedure just long enough to scold, "Come on now. Buck up. This couldn't possibly hurt that much!" The provider had contradicted and criticized the patient for feeling what she felt. His comment conveyed the message that her feelings were wrong, and this left her feeling humiliated and angry. His comment motivated her to find a new dentist.

This older adult's experience with her dentist provides a context for this next point: At least 70% of all healthcare-related lawsuits are related to poor communication (Phelps & Hassed, 2012). When an older adult feel deserted, devalued, and disempowered, or the information was provided in a rushed, non-caring, disrespectful manner, feelings are sometimes hurt and, if not resolved, can lead to litigation. When this occurs, a sincere apology from the provider (which takes responsibility and conveys regret) can help reduce anger and blame. It can also help to restore trust, repair the professional relationship, and decrease the risk of a malpractice lawsuit (Robbennolt, 2009).

## PROVIDING EMOTIONAL SUPPORT: HELPING WORDS, HARMFUL WORDS

Within the aging services network, it is common for providers to offer encouragement and emotional support to older adults. Emotional support can be understood as providing care and concern—especially at those times when the older adult is experiencing stress (see Chapter 7 *Person-Centered Communication and Stress*).

The older adult who feels emotionally supported often feels more comfortable and more cared for—as if he or she matters. The older adult who feels emotionally unsupported often feels more discomfort, disinterest, and also feels uncared for—as if he or she does not matter.

Emotional support is frequently conveyed via acknowledging feelings, mindful listening, demonstrating empathy and understanding, and by legitimizing and validating the emotions of the older adult. Lack of emotional support often stems from feelings of not being listened to, and/or having personal feelings criticized, dismissed, or invalidated, and from feeling unseen, unheard and/or misunderstood.

The comments from providers who claim they "totally understand" what the older adult is feeling or going through are often unhelpful and can sometimes be harmful. In an interview for this book, a hospice nurse shared her experience of attending the death of a teenaged patient. She reported that less than five minutes after the young boy had died—his body lying on the bed in front of the family—an apparently well-meaning relative turned to the grieving parents and said, "At least now, he's in a better place." The grief-stricken parents said nothing. Weeks later, in a follow-up visit to the family, the mother of the deceased young boy—with angry tears in her eyes—shared this, "When she made that comment, I felt like I was being stabbed in the heart. He's in a better place now? Bullcrap! Didn't she know that there is no better place than right here in my arms?"

## CONCLUDING THE PROVIDER–OLDER ADULT INTERACTION

When an older adult has a need, problem, or concern, he or she seeks out a provider hoping that this person will be able to help in some way. The provider and older adult come together for an interaction. A respectful, rapport-based professional relationship is established and sustained utilizing a person-centered communication approach. Both technical and clinical skills are used to identify and address the older adult's concerns.

When the interaction is nearing conclusion, it is helpful to ask if any questions or concerns remain. Example: "Is there anything else you'd like to ask before you leave?" or "Have we addressed all your concerns for today?"

Many times, the older adult's needs, concerns, or problems will require ongoing care—more than one visit. In such cases, it is best if at least some resolution occurs during each interaction (Tamparo & Lindh, 2008). This leaves the older adult feeling that progress is being made—feeling hopeful.

## LIST OF MAIN POINTS FOR PREVIEW AND REVIEW

### Provider Self-Test and/or Discussion Suggestions for Instructors
**Discuss:** The importance and benefits of a rapport-based professional relationship with an older adult.

**Explain:** How professional relationships develop. Be certain to address the role of rapport, connection, and communication.

**Discuss:** The philosophy of person-centered care. Identify key characteristics. Differentiate person-centered from provider-centered giving examples of each.

**List:** Several ways that rapport may be developed and deepened.

**Explain:** The process of *mirroring*, what it is used for, and how it is done.

**Discuss:** The importance of calling an individual by his or her name. Integrate the concept of *elderspeak* into your discussion.

**Define:** The concepts of *deep listening, multitasking,* and *mindfulness.* Talk about their role in the process of cultivating rapport.

**Outline:** The communication cycle. Differentiate between social and professional communication. Discuss the three-step helping interview, the communication cycle, the four modes of communication, the seven C's, and how the interaction can be brought to a close.

**Discuss:** The three types of questions and provide examples of each.

**List:** Some of the ways to enhance effective communication and some of the common barriers to effective communication.

# WEB RESOURCES

American Academy on Communication in Healthcare
http://www.aachonline.org/dnn/Home.aspx

**Person-Centered Care**
Institute for Person-Centered Care
http://ubipcc.com/
The National Communication Association
https://www.natcom.org/

# REFERENCES

Adams, C. H., & Jones, P. D. (2011). *Therapeutic communication for health professionals.* New York, NY: McGraw-Hill.

Bras, M., Dordevic, V., & Janjanin, M. (2013). Person-centered pain management – science and art. *Croatian Medical Journal, 54*(3), 296–300.

Dreher, B. B. (2001). *Communication skills for working with elders.* New York, NY: Springer Publishing Co.

Drench, M. E., Noonan, A. C., Sharby, N., & Ventura, S. H. (2012). *Psychosocial aspects of health care.* Upper Saddle River, NJ: Pearson.

Hart, V. A. (2010). *Patient-provider communications: Caring to listen.* Sudbury, MA: Jones and Bartlett Publishers.

Meldrum, H. (August 2005). Counseling patients on ACM medications: synthesizing communication and rhetorical theory. *Alternative & Complementary Therapies,* 191–196.

Mish, F. C. (Ed.). (2009). *Merriam-Webster's collegiate dictionary.* Springfield, MS: Merriam-Webster, Inc.

Moses, G. (2005). Complementary and alternative medicine use in the elderly [geriatric therapeutics]. *Journal of Pharmaceutical Practice Research, 35,* 63–68.

Phelps, K., & Hassed, C. (2012). *Communication with patients.* Kindle edition. Chatswood, NSW: Elsevier, Australia.

Robbennolt, J. K. (2009). Apologies and medical error. *Clinical Orthopedics and Related Research*, 467(2), 376–382.

Spitzberg, B. H., & Cupach, W. R. (1984). *Interpersonal communication competence.* Beverly Hills, CA: Sage.

Tamparo, C. D., & Lindh, W. Q. (2008). *Therapeutic communications for healthcare.* Clifton Park, New York: Thompson Delmar Learning.

Watzlawick, P. (1967). *The pragmatics of human communication.* New York, NY: W. W. Norton & Co.

CHAPTER 5

# Person-Centered Communication: Ageism—the Core Problem

*Ageism is as odious as racism and sexism.*

*Claude Pepper*

**Core Question:** What is ageism, and how does it impact the older adult, the provider–older adult relationship, and the person-centered approach to communication?

**Keywords:** Ageism; Bigotry; Discrimination; Elder abuse; Elderspeak prejudice; Stereotype.

## INTRODUCTION

This chapter discusses the widespread, cross-cultural problem of ageism and explores its impact on the older adult, the professional relationship, and the person-centered approach to communication.

Ageism is a cross-cultural social concern, especially prevalent in the United States (Williams & Nussbaum, 2001). Ageism is the tendency to negatively stereotype older adults, to display prejudice against the elderly, and discriminate against people simply because they are older. Founded in myths, stereotypes, and language that conjures up negative images, ageist beliefs can significantly interfere with a provider's ability to communicate effectively and respectfully. At the extreme, ageism can lead to neglect, mistreatment, and abuse. As an antidote to help reduce ageism, providers are encouraged to adopt guidelines from the respect-based, person-centered approach to communication.

## AGEISM—A FORMIDABLE EXPRESSION OF BIGOTRY

The term *ageism* was coined in 1968 by Robert Butler—a Pulitzer Prize winning gerontologist who founded the National Institute on Aging. Dr. Butler described *ageism* as a process of systematic stereotyping and discrimination against people because they are old (Butler, 1969). He likened ageism to two other forms of bigotry—sexism and racism. VandenBos (2009)

*Person-Centered Communication with Older Adults*
http://dx.doi.org/10.1016/B978-0-12-420132-3.00005-2

defined *ageism* as "the tendency to be prejudiced against older adults and to negatively stereotype them" (p. 11).

> *Ageism is based on stereotypes, myths about aging, and language that conjures up negative images of older adults. Ageism is to old age as racism is to skin color and sexism is to gender. Ageist thinking is detrimental to society and can result in limited opportunities for adults. In its worst form, ageism leads to elder abuse, mistreatment, and neglect.*
>
> **Robnett and Chop (2010, p. 22)**

Ageism can significantly impact the communication process, threaten the integrity of the provider–older adult relationship, and create unnecessary and unhealthy levels of stress in the older adult.

An argument could easily be made that providers who harbor ageist attitudes violate their professional injunction to "do no harm." Nemmers (2004) issued this warning, "Conscious or unconscious ageist attitudes and stereotypes could significantly influence the cognitive and physical functioning of the elderly patient, and might possibly affect the elderly individuals' will to survive and continue living" (p. 17).

## CONCEPTUAL BASIS OF AGEISM: PREJUDICE, STEREOTYPING, DISCRIMINATION

Chapter 2 argued that each individual provider operates through a worldview—a set of assumptions, beliefs, and interpreted experiences that informs and influences attitudes and understanding of aging and older adults. One objective of this chapter is to encourage providers to cultivate a worldview of aging and older adults that fosters a respectful perspective that views each person as a unique individual.

The human brain categorizes. Apparently, this normal cognitive process functions to help make sense of personal experience by grouping objects and events based on shared and/or similar characteristics. The brain's capacity for organizing experiential data is helpful for functioning in society. But when this capacity is used for categorizing people, problems can arise that impede the process of person–centered communication.

One such problem is that when the brain assigns an individual to membership in a specific group or category (such as "old people"), it tends to perceive the person as more similar to all other members of that group and as less similar to members of a different group (such as "young people") (Nelson, 2002, p. 6). This type of categorization and labeling can give rise to stereotypes, such as "all older adults are similar." It fosters the mistaken belief that more homogeneity is present than actually exists. Contrary to widespread belief, the population of older adults is not homogeneous. It is one of the most diverse groups in society. Older adults are just as unique as younger adults.

Prejudice is "a negative attitude toward another person or group formed in advance of an experience with that person or group—it pre-judges. Prejudice includes an affective component (emotions that range from mild nervousness to hatred), a cognitive component (assumptions and beliefs about groups, including stereotypes), and a behavioral component (negative behaviors, including discrimination and violence)" (VandenBos, 2009, p. 317).

Similar to racism and sexism, ageism perceives and treats people based on stereotypes about a group. A stereotype is "a set of cognitive generalizations (e.g., beliefs, expectations) about the qualities and characteristics of the members of a particular group or social category" (VandenBos, 2009, p. 405). A sample of common ageist stereotypes include the following:

- All older adults are alike.
- The elderly are all conservative and crabby.
- Most older adults are senile.
- Older people do not enjoy sex.
- Older adults have poor memories and forget everything.
- Older adults move too slowly.

Age discrimination "occurs when individuals are treated differently because of their chronological age" (Ekerdt, 2002, p. 28). *Discrimination* is the "differential treatment of the members of different ethnic, religious, national, or other groups. Discrimination is usually the behavioral manifestation of prejudice" (VandenBos, 2009, p. 108).

Interpersonal communication between a provider and an older adult takes place within the context of a person-centered, professional relationship. During an interaction, there is nothing socially inappropriate or offensive when the provider notices the age of the individual he or she is speaking with. As Nelson (2002) reminds, "It is what we do with that information that can be destructive" (p. 3).

## ROOTS OF AGEISM

Many cultures endorse a worldview that holds elders in high esteem and views them as a collective source of accumulated wisdom birthed in a depth of mature, lived experience. This "constructive stereotype" is in contrast to that in the United States where—because beauty, youth, and vitality are so highly valued—older adults are frequently seen as nonproductive and often treated as burdensome (Loue & Sajatovic, 2008).

Ageism appears in many forms, has a variety of causes, and serves a number of functions (Nelson, 2002). Fueled by numerous myths, a powerful but misguided media, and by a language that conjures negative images of old persons, ageism could be characterized as an assault on the collective self-image, self-esteem, and self-worth of older adults. It contributes to discrimination in the workplace and in the healthcare system, and—in its most insidious form—to elder abuse.

Ageist attitudes are perpetuated in many ways. Television advertising repeatedly endorses negative stereotypes by representing older adults as forgetful, temperamental, and stubborn. Although recent improvements are encouraging, a shortage of positive elderly role models on television remains. Many jokes and comments made about growing old and the elderly perpetuate negative stereotypes about the aging process and about older persons. The greeting card industry publishes birthday cards employing humor to decry the advance of age. The lexicon is replete with ageist terms such as "old fart," "old maid," "old geezer," "old coot," "dirty old man," "old goat," "old battle ax," "old blue hair," "over the hill," and "one foot in the grave."

In addition to the preoccupation with youth and vitality by American culture, a widespread fear of death seems to exist. Since death is the ultimate outcome of the aging process—and because older adults are closer to death than younger adults—some theorists believe that ageism functions similar to a psychological defense mechanism designed to help protect against this fear. In this view, ageism is a defense that operates by creating physical, emotional, and psychological distance between younger adults and older adults in an attempt to mitigate the fear of death (Nelson, 2002; Tornstam, 2005).

Whatever the historical roots and contemporary causes of an ageist attitude may be, its presence in a provider can trigger a chain reaction of toxic consequences. At its worst, these consequences can negatively impact the physical, emotional, and mental health of the older adult, derail the professional relationship, and contaminate the person-centered communication process.

## CONSEQUENCES OF AGEISM

The stereotyping of an older adult is dehumanizing and objectifying. Often—as a consequence of stereotyping—the older person is no longer seen as a unique human being, but instead is viewed more like a ludicrous caricature formed of the bits and pieces of collective fears, ignorance, distortions, exaggerations, and sweeping overgeneralizations.

An older adult, once objectified, can more easily be denied rights and opportunities. Viewing people as objects increases the probability they may be mistreated and/or suffer abuse. Ageist beliefs can significantly interfere with a provider's ability to communicate effectively and respectfully. Touhy and Jett (2011) provide this example:

> If the nurse believes that all older people have memory problems, or are unable to learn or process information, he or she will be less likely to engage in conversation, provide appropriate health information, or treat the person with respect and dignity (p. 82).

## AGEISM IS AN ASSAULT ON RESPECT AND DIGNITY

Hart (2010) emphasizes that effective communication with older adults is based on respect. Providers who show respect for older adults convey the message that they hold such persons in high esteem or regard—a healthy and constructive message that supports the individual and invites honest communication.

There are many ways a provider can demonstrate respect. Being courteous and attentive are core aspects of showing respect. These behaviors evince dignity and interest. Listening is also a very important form of showing respect (Sung, Kim, & Torres-Gil, 2010). Framing communication according to the guidelines suggested by the "seven C's" (discussed in Chapter 3) is another method. Expressing interest in the older adult's personal history as well as presenting concerns is another way to communicate respect.

Paying attention to the older adult when he or she is speaking is critically important. Individuals engaged in conversation can nearly always sense if the listener is truly paying attention. The provider who is a mindful listener makes a sincere effort to keep his or her eyes on the speaker as much as possible—not a chart, laptop computer, smartphone, or tablet—or, if necessary, excuses themselves once the interaction is complete to finish charting. This shows respect.

During a provider–older adult interaction, if the older adult is lying in bed or sitting in a wheelchair, the provider should position him or herself at the eye level of the individual rather than talking over a side rail or standing above them (Touhy & Jett, 2011). This demonstrates respect. During an encounter with a provider, the older adult wants to be seen for who she or he is—a unique individual. To do so is to show respect. During the interaction, the older adult is paying attention—listening for the content of what is being communicated—and taking note of how she or he is being treated.

The provider's task is simple: Treat each older adult with respect, and keep the needs of the older person as the central focus of the interaction. Utilizing appropriate clinical skills to identify the older adult's concerns, problems, or needs and attempting to constructively address them is also showing respect. Purtilo and Haddad (2002) advise, "The secret to respectful interaction with older people is to keep their age-related problems in mind while concentrating on their individuality" (p. 306).

Overall, the provider practicing a person-centered approach to service delivery can demonstrate respect by viewing the older adult as a unique individual, demonstrating genuine concern and caring, and by listening and paying attention. The older adult who feels seen, heard, understood, cared for—and as if they genuinely matter—is an older adult who probably feels respected.

## Example of Disrespect

This is an excerpt from an interview with a patient's daughter.

"I walked into the hospital room along with some caregivers where my mother was lying in bed. She was alert but didn't talk much. Ignoring my mother, one of the caregivers started talking with me and another staff person about the progression of her illness. As the conversation continued in this way—caregivers talking about my mother as if she was not in the room—my mother looked at me and covered her ears. No one but me even noticed her. I understood what she was trying to say and immediately escorted everyone out of the room. I realized that my mother's hearing was fully intact even though she wasn't saying anything. I fought back the tears as I also realized how rude, inappropriate, and disrespectful it had been for the staff to talk about the progression of her illness in front of my mother as if she wasn't there."

## ELDERSPEAK

What's in a name? Respect, for one thing. During the initial encounter, providers are advised to call the older adult by his or her surname. After that, ask the older adult how he or she wants to be addressed. Unless an older adult prefers to be called by something other than his or her given name, doing so could be construed as an expression of ageism and a sign of disrespect. For example, referring to an older adult as "honey" or "sweetie" during an interaction is not person-centered. Considered a form of *elderspeak*, it is patronizing and condescending. It tends to devalue the uniqueness of the individual and carries a negative connotation.

Just as there are many different ways of demonstrating respect for an older adult, there are also numerous ways of showing disrespect. One of the most common expressions of disrespect is termed *elderspeak*. Elderspeak refers to the tendency of some individuals to inappropriately adjust their speech patterns when communicating with older adults. Resembling a form of "baby talk," elderspeak is an expression of ageism—a problem rampant within the network of aging services providers, especially in hospitals, clinics, skilled care nursing facilities, and the assisted-living industry.

Elderspeak is a style of speech characterized by the use of simplified vocabulary, a higher pitch, an increasing volume, singsong intonation, and use of endearing or diminutive terms such as "cutie" (Touhy & Jett, 2011). It is an all too common style of speaking with older adults that has significant potential for negative consequences (Williams, Kemper, & Hummert, 2004).

*Once when I was walking back to the exam room, the aide said, "So how are we today?" I just smiled and said, "Fine." But, I thought to myself, I'm not a "we" and I'm not "fine."*

**Anonymous patient**

Elderspeak is also characterized by the inappropriate use of pronouns. Examples: "How are we today, Mrs. Smith?" "Are we ready for our bath?" "Do we need some help getting dressed this morning?" (Hart, 2010). A much better way to address older adults is to ask, "Mrs. Smith, are you ready for your bath? or "Do you need help getting dressed?"

## ELDER SPEAK: COMPARE AND CONTRAST

Mary, a medication aide at an assisted living facility, is assigned to remind 87-year-old Mrs. Jones when it's time to take her pain medications. It is time for her next dose. Here are two versions of what Mary could say.

**A.** "Hello Dear. It's time for us to take our medicine." Mrs. Jones takes her medicine. Mary responds, "Good girl!"

**B.** "Hello Mrs. Jones. It's time for your next dose of medicine." Mrs. Jones takes her medicine. Mary responds, "I'll come back when it's time for your next dose."

Question: If you were Mrs. Jones, which version would you find more respectful?

Most providers probably do not realize how often they use elderspeak or understand the negative messages conveyed when they do (Talerico, 2005). The provider using elderspeak may be well-intentioned, but for the recipient, this style of speaking is equivalent to being treated as a child and implies incompetence. It is disrespectful, demeaning, demoralizing, and can have negative physical health consequences (Williams et al., 2004). Talerico (2005) warns that "the messages inherent in elderspeak may unknowingly reinforce dependency and engender isolation and depression, contributing to the spiral of decline in physical, cognitive, and functional status" (p. 14).

Harmful ageist stereotypes are perpetuated and reinforced when older adults are repeatedly spoken to in the patronizing manner of elderspeak. Older adults who are repeatedly exposed to elderspeak are at risk for internalizing and accepting these ageist beliefs as accurate and valid. When this occurs, "negative age stereotypes can become a self-fulfilling prophecy" (Savundranayagam & Ryan, 2008, p. 52). Hart (2010) argues that older adults exposed to frequent elder speak "may respond with dependent behavior, lower self-esteem, frustration, and little respect for the healthcare provider" (p. 170).

### Example of Elderspeak Versus the Person-Centered Approach

Mr. Brown, an 83-year-old new resident in an assisted living facility, is walking back to his apartment, #116. He mistakenly tries to enter the wrong apartment, #119. A facility staff person observes Mr. Brown struggling to fit his key into the wrong door and decides to intervene. The following scenarios illustrate different approaches the staff person might take. In the first scenario, the staff person uses elderspeak. In the second, she uses a respectful, person-centered approach.

**A.** "Mr. Brown, where do we think we're going? That's not our room." Mr. Brown continues to try and enter the wrong apartment. The staff person responds, "We really are confused, aren't we?" Taking his hand without asking, the staff person comments, "Come on now Honey. Our room is right across the hall."

**B.** "Mr. Brown, because all these doors look alike, it's easy to get them mixed up. Lots of residents do. This is apartment #119. Your apartment is #116 and is right across the hall. May I open the door for you?"

Elderspeak can be viewed as the polar opposite of the person-centered approach to communication. Because it is a dehumanizing and objectifying manner of interacting with older adults, it could place some individuals at greater risk for abuse.

## ELDER ABUSE

The negative stereotypes that lead to ageist attitudes, language, and behavior also place older adults at greater risk of abuse. Abuse can be physical, emotional, mental, or financial. In 1987, Congress defined *elder abuse* as the domestic and institutional abuse of persons over age 60 involving physical, sexual, and emotional/psychological harm, as well as neglect, self-neglect, abandonment, and financial exploitation. Abuse can occur in the older person's home or in the home of a caregiver (domestic setting); in an assisted living, skilled care nursing, or institutional setting; or it may be self-inflicted.

Elder abuse is a crime. It constitutes a serious violation of human rights and can result in an older adult suffering loss of dignity and self-respect; emotional and psychological harm such as anxiety, depression, and posttraumatic stress disorder; severe financial loss or ruin; and physical injury, disability, or death. The National Center on Elder Abuse reports medical costs incurred due to elder abuse top $5.9 billion annually, and annual financial loss due to exploitation is estimated at $2.9 billion (http://www.ncea.aoa.gov).

The exact size of the problem is unknown, and estimates vary widely, but the fact remains: The abuse of older adults in the United States is a national disgrace. The National Center on Elder Abuse reported that the results of one study indicated between 7 and 10% of elders may suffer some abuse each year. The Administration on Aging estimates that 2.1 million older adults are victims of abuse each year (http://www.aoa.gov). The World Health Organization estimates that globally approximately 4–6% of older adults have experienced some form of abuse.

In March 2010, the Elder Justice Act (EJA) was passed. This was an important milestone. The culmination of a decades-long effort to help address the national problem of protecting vulnerable older adults, the EJA is the first federal law that specifically states that older adults have the right to be free of abuse, neglect, and exploitation.

## DETECTING AND REPORTING ELDER ABUSE

Many providers within the aging services network have completed training in the prevention, detection, and reporting of elder abuse and are classified as "mandatory reporters." If a provider is considered a mandatory reporter, he or she is required to report suspected abuse to appropriate authorities. But even with specific training, the majority of cases go undetected and unreported. It is estimated that for every reported case of elder abuse, approximately five remain unreported (www.aoa.gov).

One reason for underdetection is the reluctance of older adults to report abuse. They may feel embarrassed, humiliated, or fear retaliation. They may lack the physical and/or cognitive capacity to report, or because 90% of abusers are family members, they may choose to protect the perpetrator.

## CONCLUSION

Ageism is a widespread, cross-cultural social problem. Especially prevalent in the United States, it can be viewed as a national disgrace. This chapter was written to help providers increase awareness of ageism, elderspeak, and elder abuse and to explore how to overcome the formidable challenges they present to the person-centered approach to communication.

Ageism is the tendency to negatively stereotype older adults, to display prejudice against the elderly, and discriminate against people simply because they are older. Founded in myths, stereotypes, and language that conjures up negative images, ageism can impact the communication process, threaten the integrity of the provider–older adult relationship, and create unhealthy levels of stress in the older adult. At the extreme, ageism can lead to neglect, mistreatment, and abuse. Ageist beliefs can significantly interfere with a provider's ability to communicate effectively and respectfully. Providers who harbor ageist attitudes violate their professional injunction to "do no harm." As an antidote to help reduce ageism, these seven guidelines based on the person-centered approach to communication are suggested:

- Treat each older adult as a unique individual.
- Treat each older adult with respect, displaying genuine care and concern.
- Listen mindfully. Be attentive and courteous.
- Avoid elderspeak. Strive to recognize any personal, age-based stereotypes and attitudes and work to overcome them.
- Keep the needs of the older person as the central focus of the interaction.
- Utilize appropriate clinical skills to identify the older adult's concerns, problems, or needs and attempt to constructively address them.
- Frame communication according to the guidelines suggested by the seven "*C's*."

Ageism appears in many forms, has a variety of causes, is perpetuated in many ways, and serves a number of functions. What is the bottom line? Ageism is a dehumanizing, objectifying, demeaning, and demoralizing social problem affecting millions of people both in the United States and around the world.

There are many challenges to effective, person-centered communication. Ageism is only one. Accurate communication between providers and older adults is hindered by some of the normal physiological changes associated with the process of aging and by issues related to an increasingly diverse, multicultural population of older adults. These are some of the other challenges that will be explored in the next chapter.

## LIST OF MAIN POINTS FOR PREVIEW AND REVIEW

- Ageism is a process of systematic stereotyping and discrimination against people because they are older in years—the tendency to be prejudiced against older adults and to negatively stereotype them.
- Ageism can significantly impact the communication process, threaten the integrity of the provider–older adult relationship, and create unhealthy levels of stress in the older adult. In its worst form, ageism leads to elder abuse, mistreatment, and neglect.
- Ageism is especially prevalent in the United State and presents a formidable barrier to effective, person-centered communication.
- Ageism is based on stereotypes, myths about aging, and language that conjures up negative images of older adults.
- The stereotyping of an older adult is dehumanizing and objectifying.
- A stereotype is a set of cognitive generalizations about the qualities and characteristics of the members of a particular group or social category.
- Prejudice is a negative attitude toward another person or group formed in advance of an experience with that person or group.
- Age discrimination occurs when individuals are treated differently because of their chronological age.
- Discrimination is the differential treatment of the members of different ethnic, religious, national, or other groups.
- Contrary to widespread belief, the population of older adults is not homogeneous. It is one of the most diverse groups in society. Older adults are just as unique as younger adults.
- Some theorists believe ageism functions similar to a psychological defense mechanism designed to help protect against fear of death. In this view, ageism is a defense that operates by creating physical, emotional, and psychological distance between younger adults and older adults in an attempt to mitigate the fear of death.
- Providers who show respect for older adults convey the message that they hold such persons in high esteem or regard.
- There are many ways a provider can demonstrate respect. Some include being courteous, attentive, listening, and framing communication according to the guidelines suggested by the seven "C's."

- During an encounter with a provider, the older adult wants to be seen for who she or he is—a unique individual.
- The provider's task is simple: Treat each older adult with respect, demonstrate genuine concern and caring, and keep the needs of the older person as the central focus of the interaction. Utilize appropriate clinical skills to identify the older adult's concerns, problems, or needs and attempt to constructively address them.
- Providers are advised to call the older adult by his or her surname.
- Elderspeak refers to the tendency of some individuals to inappropriately adjust their speech patterns when communicating with older adults. Resembling a form of "baby talk," elderspeak is an expression of ageism characterized by the use of simplified vocabulary, a higher pitch, an increase in volume, singsong intonation, and use of endearing or diminutive terms such as "honey" or "cutie."
- Elderspeak is also characterized by the inappropriate use of pronouns, for example, "How are we today, Mrs. Smith?"
- Harmful ageist stereotypes are perpetuated and reinforced when older adults are repeatedly spoken to in the patronizing manner of elderspeak.
- Elderspeak is a patronizing and condescending expression of ageism. It is a disrespectful, demeaning, devaluing, and demoralizing style of communication that places the older adult at risk for increased dependency, depression, and other negative health consequences. Because it is a dehumanizing and objectifying manner of interacting with older adults, it could place some individuals at greater risk for abuse.
- Elder abuse can be physical, emotional, mental, or financial. It constitutes a serious violation of human rights and can result in an older adult suffering loss of dignity and self-respect; emotional and psychological harm such as anxiety, depression, and posttraumatic stress disorder; severe financial loss or ruin; and physical injury, disability, or death.
- Between 7 and 10% of elders may suffer some abuse each year. It is estimated that for every reported case of elder abuse, approximately five remain unreported. One reason for underdetection is the reluctance of older adults to report abuse. They may feel embarrassed, humiliated, or fear retaliation. They may lack the physical and/or cognitive capacity to report, or because 90% of abusers are family members, they may choose to protect the perpetrator.
- In March 2010, the Elder Justice Act (EJA) was passed. The EJA is the first federal law that specifically states that older adults have the right to be free of abuse, neglect, and exploitation.

## Provider Self-Test and/or Suggestions for Instructors

**Explore:** Personal feelings about growing older and about older adults.

**Define:** The key concepts of *ageism, stereotyping, prejudice*, and *discrimination*.

**Identify:** Personal stereotypes or prejudices held about older adults. Use learning methods described in Chapter 2; mental imagery techniques explained in Chapter 8; and concepts from the physics of connection explained in Chapter 10 to develop a personalized program for professional growth.

**List:** Some of the negative consequences of ageism. Discuss how ageist attitudes impact the older adult, influence the provider–older adult relationship, and their effect upon society.

**Explain:** How ageism might function as a psychological defense against the fear of death and dying.

**Describe:** Some of ways ageism is perpetuated in the American culture and discuss how it might be reduced.

**Discuss:** The concept of *ageism* in terms of the professional duty to "do no harm."

**Explain:** The role that dehumanizing behavior and objectifying stereotypes play in elder abuse. List several ways a provider could demonstrate respect for an older adult.

**Define:** *Elderspeak.* Provide several examples and discuss its detrimental effect on older adults.

**Discuss:** The prevalence of elder abuse in the United States. Describe the different types of abuse and their negative impact on older adults and upon the overall economy. Identify reasons why elder abuse is often underdetected and underreported.

# WEB RESOURCES

Administration on aging
   http://www.aoa.gov/
National Adult Protective Services Association
   http://www.napsa-now.org/
National Center Elder Abuse
   http://www.ncea.aoa.gov
World Health Organization
   http://www.who.int/ageing/projects/elder_abuse/en/

## Journals

Journal of Elder Abuse & Neglect
   http://www.tandfonline.com/loi/wean20#.VHOVfJXF-zQ

Explores clinical and ethical issues surrounding the abuse and neglect of older people.

## REFERENCES

Butler, R. (1969). Ageism: another form of bigotry. *The Gerontologist, 9*(4), 243–246.

Ekerdt, D. J. (Ed.). (2002). *Encyclopedia of aging.* New York, NY: Thomson Gale.

Hart, J. (2010). Teaching humanism in medical training. *Alternative and Complementary Therapies, 17*(1), 9–13.

Loue, S., & Sajatovic, M. (Eds.). (2008). *Encyclopedia of aging and public health.* New York, NY: Springer.

Nelson, T. D. (Ed.). (2002). *Ageism: Stereotyping and prejudice against older persons.* Cambridge, MA: MIT Press.

Nemmers, T. M. (2004). The influence of ageism and ageist stereotypes on the elderly. *Physical & Occupational Therapy in Geriatrics, 22*(4), 11–20.

Purtilo, R., & Haddad, A. (2002). *Health professional and patient interaction.* New York, NY: W.B. Saunders Company.

Robnett, R. H., & Chop, W. C. (2010). *Gerontology for the health care professional.* Sudbury, MA: Jones and Bartlett Publishers.

Savundranayagam, M. Y., & Ryan, E. B. (2008). Social psychological aspects of communications and aging. *Annual Review of Applied Linguistics, 28*, 51–72.

Sung, K. T., Kim, B. J., & Torres-Gil, F. (2010). Respectfully treating the elderly: affective and behavioral ways of American young adults. *Educational Gerontology, 36*, 127–147.

Talerico, K. A. (2005). Enhancing communication with older adults overcoming elderspeak. *Journal of Psychosocial Nursing, 43*(5), 12–16.

Tornstam, L. (2005). *Gerotranscendence: A developmental theory of positive aging.* New York, NY: Springer Publishing Company.

Touhy, T. A., & Jett, K. F. (2011). *Ebersole & Hess' toward healthy aging: Human needs and nursing response.* St. Louis, MO: Elsevier, Mosby.

VandenBos, G. R. (Ed.). (2009). *APA college dictionary of psychology.* Washington, DC: American Psychological Association.

Williams, K., Kemper, S., & Hummert, M. L. (2004). Enhancing communication with older adults: overcoming elderspeak. *Journal of Gerontological Nursing, 30*(10), 17–25.

Williams, A., & Nussbaum, J. F. (2001). *Intergenerational communication across the lifespan.* Mahwah, NJ: Lawrence Erlbaum Associates.

# CHAPTER 6

# Person-Centered Communication: Age-Related Changes, Cultural Challenges, and Difficult Conversations

*Never take a person's dignity: It is worth everything to them, and nothing to you.*

*Frank X. Barron*

**Core Question:** How can the person-centered communication approach assist the provider when discussing sensitive issues with older adults, when interacting with older adults from another culture, and/or when interacting with older adults suffering from hearing loss, aphasia, or dementia?

**Keywords:** Advanced directives; Age-related hearing loss; Alzheimer's disease; Aphasia; Confidentiality; Dementia; Ethnocentrism; HIPPA; Informed consent; Presbycusis.

## INTRODUCTION

Chapter 4 discussed common barriers to person-centered communication. Communication can also be hindered by numerous other challenges—far too many to explore in this book. These challenges include discussion of informed consent, confidentiality and privacy, advanced directives, sharing "bad news," personal relationship and family issues, and end-of-life concerns. Other challenges include issues associated with provider–older adult cultural differences and numerous physiological changes common to the aging process that can affect communication.

This chapter discusses informed consent, confidentiality, advanced directives, multicultural challenges, and three common age-related changes—hearing loss, aphasia, and cognitive impairments. It discusses how these challenges and changes can impact the exchange of information, the professional relationship, and influence the process of interpersonal communication.

*Person-Centered Communication with Older Adults*
http://dx.doi.org/10.1016/B978-0-12-420132-3.00006-4

## PROVIDERS, OLDER ADULTS, AND THE EXCHANGE OF INFORMATION

Providers and older adults exchange various types of information. This includes information about health, informed consent, privacy, confidentiality, and medications; lifestyle concerns such as residence, relationships, diet, exercise, transportation, and safety; insurance, financial and legal information; and other information related to psychosocial needs, problems, and concerns.

Because the process of how information is shared is just as important as the content itself, Chapters 3 and 4 recommended providers form a rapport-based relationship, use person-centered communication guided by the principles referred to as the seven 'C's' and three special 'C's' to provide encouragement and to identify and attempt to resolve the older adult's presenting concerns. This recommendation becomes even more appropriate when discussing sensitive or emotionally laden topics.

## INFORMED CONSENT

Within the field of health care, the informed consent agreement is one of the most central and frequently discussed concepts (Kukla, 2009). Used in virtually all health care institutions within the United States, they are written documents designed to help govern patient–provider interactions (Purtilo & Haddad, 2002). Jonsen, Siegler, and Winsdale (2002) defined informed consent as "the willing acceptance of a medical intervention by a patient after adequate disclosure by the physician of the nature of the intervention, its risks and benefits, and also its alternatives with their risks and benefits" (p. 52).

The purpose of an informed consent agreement is to provide enough information for the patient so that he or she can make reasoned decisions about the course of treatment (Purtilo & Haddad, 2002). Cultural factors and language differences can present significant challenges to securing informed consent. Another significant challenge to entering into an informed consent agreement is the use of professional jargon. As Jonsen et al. (2002) explained,

> Physicians should avoid technical terms, attempt to translate statistical data into everyday probabilities, ask whether the patient understands the information, and invite questions. The comprehension of the patient is fully as important as the provision of the information (p. 53).

The use of jargon can be intimidating to many patients. Many older adults may feel embarrassed to admit it, so they often do not say anything or raise questions. It is the provider's responsibility to make sure the older adult understands to what he or she is consenting. As Fremgen (2006) points out, for the informed consent to be given, the patient must understand what they are signing. This is where accurate communication becomes so important. An informed consent agreement is arrived at via an ongoing process of collaborative, person-centered communication and shared decision-making. The discussion of informed consent should be conducted in layperson's terms and understanding should be frequently assessed. Some form of the communications process described above is both an ethical obligation and a legal requirement in all 50 states (AMA Code of Medical Ethics). An informed consent agreement is not just something to be "obtained" nor simply another medical form that the patient is required to sign. An informed consent agreement develops out of ongoing, respectful, person-centered communication between the patient and provider.

## CONFIDENTIALITY

The cornerstone of ethical service delivery, especially in health care services, is the obligation to maintain patient confidentiality (Rosner, 2006). The Hippocratic Oath specifically instructs the physician not to disclose a patient's private information (Yang & Kombarakaran, 2006). When patients seek the services of a provider, they expect quality care and confidentiality. They have the right to both (Fremgen, 2006).

Patients routinely share sensitive and potentially embarrassing personal information with their health care providers. The obligation to preserve patient confidentiality is fundamental to health care (Rogers, 2006). In 1996, under President Bush, Congress passed the Health Insurance Portability and Accountability Act (popularly known as HIPPA). The goal of HIPPA is to regulate the privacy of protected patient health information. Protected patient health information includes any information that could identify the patient. HIPPA requires that providers strictly limit the disclosure of protected patient information to the minimum amount necessary in order to render appropriate medical treatment and that such information be released only to authorized parties (Fremgen, 2006).

Preserving and protecting patient confidentiality is central to the patient–provider relationship. The methodology of delivery may seem old-fashioned, but simply discussing confidentiality with patients using a person-centered approach may prove to be one of the best ways to ensure that they remain aware of the many ways their personal health information can be protected.

## ADVANCE HEALTH CARE DIRECTIVES

The increased utilization of advance health care directives is rooted in the patient self-determination act that President Bush signed into law in 1990. As Jecker, Jonsen, and Pearlman (1997) described, this important law was enacted not only to educate patients in their legal rights to be involved in decisions affecting their health care but to encourage the widespread use of advance directives. This law mandates that all adult patients who are admitted into any health care facility receiving Medicare or Medicaid funds must be asked if they have advance health care directives or if they wish to receive information about them.

An advance health care directive is a written document that describes a person's preferences as to which life-sustaining medical interventions he or she desires or does not desire should these interventions become necessary in the future due to a medical emergency or illness and should the individual be unable or unwilling to communicate his or her preferences at that time (Fremgen, 2006). In other words it provides "directives" to health care providers in "advance" of when they are needed. This is why these types of orders are referred to as advance directives. The term advance directive is a general term used when referring to a living will and/or a durable power of attorney. Advance health care directives are one expression of the concept of patient self-determination. Pautex, Herrman, and Zulian (2008) reported that some studies have shown that most patients are eager to talk about end-of-life care with their physicians. They caution that for advance directives to be used effectively, they should be viewed as a process of ongoing communication, not just another form to be filled out. Providers who enjoy a rapport-based professional relationship with their clients often find this conversation less challenging.

## CULTURAL BARRIERS

Misunderstandings are commonplace, even when a provider and older adult speak the same language and share a common cultural background. Interacting with an older adult with a different cultural background increases the possibility for misunderstandings. Culturally diverse older adults may differ on issues such as the meaning of illness, the decision-making process, or concerns related to authority, respect, and control. Robnett and Chop (2010) remind, "As providers, it is our responsibility to be aware of and respect cultural factors, and to provide service that is consistent and compatible with personal beliefs" (p. 265).

The provider should be aware of his or her own tendency toward *ethnocentrism*. Ethnocentrism "is a belief in the superiority of one's culture or ethnic group" (Drench, Noonan, Sharby, & Ventura, 2012, p. 41). It is a cultural bias. The provider interacting with an older adult from a different cultural background is advised to avoid the tendency to interpret and judge the older adults behavior through the lens of the cultural to which he or she belongs. It is also important to remember that each person is a unique individual. Just because an individual is a member of a particular culture does not necessarily mean that person will adhere to the same beliefs, customs, or traditions commonly associated with that culture (Salimbene, 2000).

## SUGGESTIONS FOR CROSS-CULTURAL COMMUNICATION

- Keep the older adult as the focus of attention, not any perceived cultural differences.
- Do not treat the older adult in the same way you would want to be treated. Do not make assumptions. Do not jump to conclusions based on your own culture and belief systems. When in doubt, ask. Do not discount or belittle different beliefs.
- Providers who work within a particular cultural community different from their own would greatly benefit from seeking further information, education, and experience specific to that culture (Tamparo & Lindh, 2008).
- To effectively communicate with any ethnic group, providers need to familiarize themselves with the common cultural beliefs and values of the group. Recognize and respect the cultures nonverbal mannerisms and gestures.
- Allow sufficient time. Try not to rush the client.
- Consider using a cultural brokering service or interpreter able to interpret the client's language and specific cultural nuances, as well as the health care culture's terminology (Tamparo & Lindh, 2008).

## AGE-RELATED HEARING LOSS AND PERSON-CENTERED COMMUNICATION

During an interaction, the ability of providers and older adults to effectively communicate is largely dependent on the capacity to hear. Diminished hearing capacity can significantly affect an older adult's ability to communicate with a provider (Nussbaum, Pecchioni, Robinson, & Thompson, 2000). Age-related hearing loss can impact nearly every aspect of service delivery (Wallhagen, 2010).

Hearing loss (presbycusis) refers to the gradual loss of hearing that occurs in most individuals as they grow older. The third most prevalent chronic condition of American older adults, it is the foremost communicative disorder affecting this population (National Institute on Deafness and other Communication Disorders, 2014; Robnett & Chop, 2010; Touhy & Jett, 2011).

The World Health Organization (2015) estimates that 33% of the global population of older adults aged 65 and older suffer from disabling hearing loss (www.who.int/mediacentre/factsheets/fs300/en/). For those aged 75 and older, prevalence of hearing impairment increases to 50% (Beers, 2004; National Institute on Deafness and other Communication Disorders, 2014).

## CAUSES OF AGE-RELATED HEARING LOSS

There are many physical and medical causes for age-related hearing loss. The auditory system changes as a consequence of the aging process. Changes to the inner and middle ear are common. Alterations can also occur along the nerve pathway that runs from the ear to brain. Deterioration of the auditory system can lead to changes in hearing sensitivity and also to a decline in the processing of speech stimuli (Ekerdt, 2002).

Various medical conditions (such as high blood pressure or diabetes) and certain medications can also play a role in hearing loss. Long-term exposure to noise is another common factor. Most older adults have some combination of age-related hearing loss and noise-induced hearing loss (National Institute on Deafness and Other Communication Disorders, 2014).

## EXPERIENCE OF HEARING LOSS

Although hearing loss occurs in both genders, men tend to experience loss of high frequencies more frequently than women. As a consequence of losing the ability to hear higher frequencies, it may be more difficult for the older adult to distinguish between certain consonants, such as C, D, F, K, P, S, and T. This can result in misunderstandings and misinterpretations. For example, the older adult may hear "bone" when the speaker said "stone." (Beers, 2004, p. 474).

Generally speaking, age-related hearing loss has a greater impact on a person's ability to hear higher pitched sounds than lower pitched ones. This is an important distinction with practical applications. For example, women tend to have higher pitched voices than men. If a female provider is aware that an older adult suffers from hearing loss, and if the provider makes whatever reasonable accommodations are called for, but the older adult is still having difficulty understanding the provider, then—because men tend to have a lower pitched voice—it may prove helpful to involve a male provider if possible.

Age-related hearing loss can make it more difficult for an older adult to understand and follow a provider's advice, instructions, or recommendations. The older adult with a hearing impairment may feel less confident in his or her ability to communicate effectively. Lack of confidence can reduce likelihood of initiating conversation or asking providers for clarification if confused (Hummert, Wieman, & Nussbaum, 1994).

Many older adults with age-related hearing loss are not aware they have it or tend to underestimate the degree of its impact on communication. They might nod and smile—giving the impression they understand when they do not. They may frequently say "what?" or request the provider to repeat comments. Questions might be answered incorrectly based on what the older adult thought was said.

There are many situations where the lack of information or misunderstanding could place an older adult at increased risk of harm, for example, medication instructions.

### Example: Medication Instructions

A female pharmacist is waiting for a customer, Mrs. Baker—an older adult with age-related hearing loss. The pharmacist has a higher pitched voice and is aware Mrs. Baker may have some difficulty understanding her. The pharmacist does not assume a problem exists—she simply recognizes the possibility. No other pharmacists are currently available.

Mrs. Baker is at the pharmacy to pick up new medication her doctor prescribed. The pharmacist describes the purpose of the medication to her providing a detailed explanation regarding proper dosage, frequency, whether or not to take with food, possible side-effects, and potential contraindications and/or reactions with other medications. She is not certain Mrs. Baker fully understands all this information, so she decides to use the teach-back method and have Mrs. Baker repeat the instructions back to her.

In her own words, Mrs. Baker repeats what she was told and demonstrates accurate understanding of the pharmacist's instructions. The pharmacist feels confident that Mrs. Baker understands the instructions and sends her on her way with new medicine in hand, along with a printed copy of all important information.

## THE TEACH-BACK TECHNIQUE

In the preceding example, the pharmacist used the teach-back method to check for customer understanding. Teach-back techniques have wide applications and are especially helpful to confirm an older adult's understanding of the information provided during an interaction with a health care provider.

Teach-back techniques involve asking the older adult to explain—in his or her own words—what he or she has been told. Example: A health care provider could pose a question such as, "I want to make sure I explained these instructions to you clearly. If you were going to instruct your wife on how to take this medicine, what would you tell her?" Use of teach-back techniques by physicians has been associated with improved patient outcomes (Harwood et al., 2012, p. 23).

When misunderstanding about health care-related information occurs, the cost can be high for the older adult patient, the physician, and society. For the older adult, misunderstanding can lead to noncompliance with treatment recommendations, adverse outcomes, and increased dissatisfaction with the provider. Health care providers who fail to check for accurate understanding are at an increased risk of a malpractice claim (Kemp, Floyd, McCord-Duncan, & Lang, 2008, p. 24). Providers have no real way of knowing what or how much of the information that was shared was understood unless they ask the older adult. The teach-back technique offers a simple method for confirming that the information offered matches the information understood.

## GENERAL RECOMMENDATIONS FOR PROVIDERS

Referring once again to the example above, the pharmacist did not prejudge the customer or the situation. She did not assume a problem existed, but she remained aware of the possibility and took appropriate action. Some older adults with age-related hearing loss will need a provider to speak louder, but not all. The best course of action is not to assume but to remain vigilant and let circumstances dictate what may or may not be appropriate. When in doubt, it is always permissible (and professional) to simply ask.

Sometimes lowering voice pitch may help. Slowing down the rate of speech may also prove helpful, but it should not be slowed enough to sound like the condescending elderspeak described in the previous chapter. Although older adults may have difficulty hearing, this does not imply that they need to be talked to as if they also have diminished cognitive capacity (Robnett & Chop, 2010).

Here are some general suggestions that may prove helpful when interacting with an older adult with hearing loss:

- Treat each person with respect and as a unique individual.
- Avoid the tendency to pre-judge.
- Try and determine if hearing is better in one ear than the other, and if so, position yourself appropriately.
- Ask the older adult what helps him or her to best hear.
- Face the older adult when speaking. Make sure he or she can see your face and mouth.
- Ask the older adult if he or she is able to hear and understand you.
- Focus on addressing the older adult's needs, concerns, or problems.
- Speak clearly, not slowly. If you need to speak more slowly, slow down only a little. Keep your hands away from your mouth.
- If necessary, speak more loudly but avoid shouting.
- Frame communication according to the guidelines offered by the ten C's.
- Check for understanding. Use the teach-back method if necessary and appropriate. If misunderstood, try again using different words.
- When topics are changed, preface the change by stating the topic.
- Be mindful of environmental noise: other people talking, music playing in background, outside sounds of construction, building and yard maintenance, etc.
- Reduce or eliminate background noise when possible.
- Move to a quieter location.
- Ask for the assistance of another provider if necessary.

## APHASIA

Aphasia is a communication disorder that results from brain damage, most commonly the result of a stroke or head trauma, but it may be due to other causes as well. Aphasia does not affect the older adult's intelligence, but it does impede the capacity to communicate—most notably the person's ability to speak and understand others. Writing and reading may also be affected.

There are different types of aphasia that can present with varying degrees of severity. These factors determine whether the older adult is left with little or no ability to talk, the capacity for fragmented speech only, or a type of speech that is fluent but devoid of meaning (Touhy & Jett, 2011). The following section lists suggestions providers can use to improve communication with older adults experiencing aphasia.

## SUGGESTIONS FOR COMMUNICATING WITH OLDER ADULTS WITH APHASIA

- Avoid the tendency to pre-judge. Treat each individual with respect and as a unique and intelligent adult.
- Face the individual and speak clearly.
- Avoid use of patronizing elderspeak. Talk to him or her as if he or she understands.
- Be patient. Focus on addressing the person's needs, concerns, or problems.
- Make increased use of the closed-end type of questions—that can be answered with a single word. Ask one question at a time and wait for a response. Repeat and/or rephrase as needed.
- Provide ample time for the individual who appears to be struggling to complete his or her thoughts. Resist the tendency to quickly jump in and complete his or her sentences or guess at the meaning (Touhy & Jett, 2011).
- Pay close attention to the individual's use of nonverbal communication—facial expressions, gestures, posture, and overall body tension/relaxation—as an aid to understanding.
- If the individual cannot respond verbally, ask him or her to respond nonverbally such as nodding the head "yes" or "no." Other possibilities include blinking eyes once for "yes" and twice for "no" or raising the right index finger (or foot) for "yes" and the left index finger (or foot) for "no."
- Tell the individual if you can't understand what he or she is communicating. If you understand part of what was said, repeat back the parts you were able to understand so that the person at least feels partially understood and so he or she can avoid unnecessary repetition.
- Employ objects in the immediate environment as visual cues.
- If appropriate and available, employ communication augmentation devices. These can range from the use of simple paper and pencil, communication books, and story boards to electronic speech-generating devices. Apps are readily available that allow older adults to use their phones, computers, and tablets to function as augmentation devices by using pictures, symbols, letters, and words to create messages (The American Speech-Language-Hearing Association, 2012).

- Ask the person if he or she is able to understand you.
- Frame communication according to the guidelines offered by the ten C's.
- When topics are changed, preface the change by stating the topic.
- Reduce or eliminate background noise when possible. Move to a quieter location if necessary.

## COMMUNICATION WITH OLDER ADULTS WITH COGNITIVE IMPAIRMENTS

Many of the age-related changes that lead to cognitive impairment are associated with a gradual and steady decline in working memory—that part of the brain responsible for temporarily storing and processing the information required for speaking and understanding language (Harwood et al., 2012).

There are many conditions that result in a cognitive impairment. One condition that can significantly affect interpersonal communication is dementia. *Dementia* is a term referring to conditions that result in deterioration of memory and cognitive processes that reduce an individual's ability to successfully perform the activities of daily living (Mayo Clinic, 2014).

Dementia can affect memory, speech, and communication. It can impede both receptive and expressive communication and significantly alter the way an older adult communicates. There is often difficulty with word finding, termed *anomia*. People with dementia may use nonsensical words. Focus and concentration is frequently and severely compromised. Mental wandering is common.

Memory loss can range from mild to extreme. The older adult with dementia may talk about seemingly unrelated topics. He or she may seem to mix past, present, and future. As a result of these and other changes, providers may feel frustrated and stressed when attempts to communicate are not as successful as hoped.

People with dementia make up about one-quarter of all older adult hospital patients, about one-half of all skilled care nursing residents, and more than 40% of all assisted living residents (Alzheimer's Association, 2014). The most common form of dementia is Alzheimer's disease. More than five million older American adults have Alzheimer's, which accounts for 60–80% of all cases of dementia (Harwood et al., 2012).

Described as the sixth leading cause of death in the United States, Alzheimer's affects approximately one in nine older adults or 11% of the older adult population (Alzheimer's Association, 2014). Older adults with Alzheimer's disease and other forms of dementia pose considerable communication challenges.

Alzheimer's disease is caused by damage to the brain's nerve cells. This damage can lead to a decline in memory, changes in behavior, and confused thinking. During the course of the disease, the damage to the brain's nerve cells eventually interferes with a person's ability to complete even the most basic of human functions such as swallowing. Ultimately fatal, in the end-stage individuals are bed-bound and require around-the-clock care (Alzheimer's Association, 2014).

Some of the most common symptoms and behaviors observed in older adults suffering from Alzheimer's disease, as described by the Mayo clinic (2014), include the following:

- Repeating questions and statements without awareness they have been said or asked before
- Forgetting recent, previous conversations
- Forgetting names of common items
- Frequently losing and misplacing personal belongings
- Mixing up words, word-finding difficulty, making up words
- Mixing up sequence and time
- Trouble with planning and solving problems
- Forgetting how to complete simple tasks, for example, inserting a key in a lock, unzipping a zipper, or dialing a phone number
- Being unable to tell time, read, or complete simple math
- Eventually forgetting the names of family members

The brain changes that occur as a result of Alzheimer's can also affect the way an older adult feels and cause some to experience the following:

- Depression and anxiety
- Disrupted sleep cycles
- Distrust and social withdrawal
- Disorientation and wandering

The incidence of Alzheimer's disease and other dementias is higher in women than in men. This may be because women tend to live longer than men, and age is the greatest known risk factor.

Appearances to the contrary, even in late-stage dementia, the individual may understand more than is apparent and can still benefit from the provider's caring, compassionate communication. For older adults with dementia, it can be very challenging to express themselves in ways others can understand, yet the need to connect and communicate remains. Despite impediments to memory and communication, the cognitively challenged older adult needs to be seen, heard, and treated as a unique and valued individual.

During interactions with an older adult who has a cognitive impairment such as dementia, the provider should be sensitive to the possibility that the individual may feel embarrassed, frustrated, and/or frightened. No matter how seemingly nonsensical, it is essential for the provider to believe that the person with dementia is attempting to communicate meaningfully and to demonstrate that belief to the individual by making the expressed effort to understand him or her.

One of the most helpful behaviors the provider can do is to treat everything the older adult says as an attempt to share something important. Because the individual with dementia cannot change his or her communication, the provider must change his or hers (Touhy & Jett, 2011). The single most important factor for a provider to remember when interacting with an older adult suffering from Alzheimer's is that behind the disease is a unique and valuable individual.

## SUGGESTIONS FOR COMMUNICATING WITH OLDER ADULTS WITH ALZHEIMER'S

- Prior to meeting with an older adult with Alzheimer's, it may prove helpful to first review the information on neurocardiology explained in Chapter 9, especially the section *Heart-Focused Practical Applications for the Provider*. This explains how providers can psychologically prepare for potentially challenging interactions.
- Treat each older adult with respect and as a unique and valuable human being.
- Introduce yourself. Explain why you are there. When you reach out to shake hands, observe his or her response to touch.
- If the person does not want to talk, if possible, come back another time.
- Sit closely and face the person at eye level.
- Use a patient, soft, and positive communicative tone when speaking to reduce likelihood of agitation. Avoid speaking too slowly (Harwood et al., 2012).
- Use multiple ways of communication (gestures, touch) and note the person's response to different approaches.
- Reduce distractions to a minimum.
- When providing instructions, give one-step directions.

- Provide encouraging and affirming statements. If you observe problem behaviors—for example, if an older woman with dementia keeps pushing you away when you attempt to comb her hair—acknowledge the feelings that the person seems to be expressing ("It seems like you don't want me to comb your hair.") (Harwood et al., 2012, p. 30).
- Allow ample time for a response to questions.
- Use gestures to demonstrate what you want the individual to do—for example, put a footstool in front of the person, point to it, touch it and say, "Please put your feet here."
- If time confusion is apparent, try to identify what time frame, past, present, or future, the person is experiencing at the moment.
- Do not try to force the person to the present. Go to where the person is framing your message according to the principles of the ten C's.
- If you are unable to understand the person's communication, try to find a common theme in the parts you were able to understand—what meaningful connection is there between apparently disparate topics? Happiness? Fear? Grief? Search for meaning.
- Recognize the individual's feelings. Respect and respond to them. Provide emotional care.
- Show interest through body posture, facial expression, nodding, and eye contact. Assume a pleasant, relaxed attitude.
- When communicating with older adults suffering from dementia, try using simple right-branching sentences, and observe whether that seems to help. A right-branching sentence is a statement where the main clause is followed by a subordinate clause. Example: "Sit down, and you won't miss your favorite TV show." The left-branching sentence has an embedded clause that interrupts the main clause: "If you don't want to miss your favorite TV show, you should sit down." It is easier for the brain to process a right-branching sentence. Right-branching sentences require less effort from the brain's working memory (Harwood et al., 2012).
- Try to avoid using sentences that begin with words and phrases such as "although," "if," "after," "before," "while," "since," "as long as," "because," and "unless." These word and phrases require the listener to remember information in the subordinate clause in order to understand the rest of the sentence. This can put a strain on working memory (Harwood et al., 2012).
- If an older adult with dementia does not understand, try repeating what was said verbatim. Verbatim repetition can help the older adult with dementia to recall what was forgotten from the original sentence. It can

reinforce the memory trace of the original statement (Harwood et al., 2012, p. 34).

- For providers involved in rendering intimate care to an older adult such as bathing, personal hygiene, or toileting, mentally place yourself in the older adult's position, and think about how vulnerable you would feel. Be gentle and kind. Take the time to learn personal preferences. Give the person your undivided attention. Do not talk about them in front of them. Let the person do as much as he or she is capable. Do not rush in and take over the entire task. Only do what the person is unable to do for themselves. You can do much to help a person retain a sense of control by breaking tasks into small steps and encouraging the older adult to do what they can (Waring, 2012).
- Be aware of your own level of stress. Create and follow a personal stress plan as explained in Chapter 7.
- When leaving, thank the older adult for his or her time, attention, and any information shared.

Above all, the provider should demonstrate genuine care and compassion using communication that respects and values the dignity and worth of the cognitively impaired older adult (Touhy & Jett, 2011).

### Exercise: What if You Had Dementia?

This exercise was inspired by Amanda Waring's highly recommended book, *The Heart of Care: Dignity in Action: Person-Centered Compassionate Elder Care* (2012).

Instructions: Using the skills of mental imagery as discussed in Chapter 8, read through the following. Use your imagination in an effort to glimpse some of the stress and challenges faced by an individual with dementia. Ideally, this will help increase your caring, understanding, and compassion for those individuals struggling with this cognitive impairment.

Imagine that your memory has steadily declined over the past few months. You can no longer conceal it. It is getting harder and harder to follow your daily routine—to do all the things you love. Often, you are unable to recall things you know you should remember—important things. Yesterday morning, you accidently left the stove burner on.

Recently, when you talk with friends and family, you frequently feel embarrassed because it is getting very difficult to find the right words and to put a cohesive sentence together. You notice many worried looks on the faces of those who know and love you, and it makes you feel anxious and afraid.

Listening to others talk, it is often difficult to make sense of what they are saying. Sometimes, you catch yourself smiling and nodding in agreement even though you are unsure of what was said. During conversations, you sometimes hear yourself utter a nonsensical word in place of the word you meant to say. You laugh it off nervously.

Your mind wanders so much, you sometimes lose track of time and feel confused about whether something happened in the past or in the present. Well-intentioned people around you frequently ask you to repeat yourself—tell you they do not understand. You feel frustrated and afraid, worried you are losing your mind.

Today, a friend mentioned how much he enjoyed his visit with you yesterday. You felt surprised and confused and had no recollection of such a visit and thought he was kidding. He was not. This has been happening more and more lately.

This afternoon you struggled to understand how to fit your key into the front door lock of the apartment where you have lived for the past 3 years. Once inside, it seemed as if certain things were missing or had been moved without your knowledge and permission. You wonder if someone is stealing things and rearranging items in your home without your permission. But who would do such things?

During the slowly moving days, you often feel lonely and want to call family members or friends but only sometimes succeed. Dialing the phone feels so complicated. Although you enjoy watching TV in the evening, most nights you struggle endlessly trying to figure out how to operate the remote control.

Lately you have felt depressed and have not been sleeping well. On occasion, you wake up during the night, find yourself in another part of your house, and cannot remember how you got there. You sit in the dark, confused, alone, and afraid. Sometimes you cry.

Providers may also find it helpful to create a similar exercise using imagination to help increase empathy for older adults suffering from age-related hearing loss and/or aphasia.

## CONCLUSION

Communication can be hindered by numerous challenges, changes, and emotionally laden issues. These challenges include discussion of informed consent, confidentiality and privacy, advanced directives, sharing "bad news," personal relationship and family issues, and end-of-life concerns. Other challenges include issues associated with provider–older adult cultural differences and numerous physiological changes common to the aging process that can affect communication.

This chapter discussed how these challenges and changes can impact the exchange of information and the professional relationship and how they can influence the process of interpersonal communication. Each older adult needs to feel seen, heard, and valued. Each can benefit from a rapport-based relationship with a respectful provider who demonstrates genuine caring and compassionate concern—a provider who utilizes a person-centered approach to communication guided by the seven regular and three special *C*'s.

The faces change, but the professional objective remains the same. No matter what the medical challenges or the cultural background of the older adult, the provider should do his or her best to identify the older adult's needs, problems, and concerns, seek to address them with sensitivity, and treat each person as a unique individual.

## LIST OF MAIN POINTS FOR PREVIEW AND REVIEW

- Communication can be hindered by numerous challenges. These include discussion of informed consent, confidentiality and privacy, advanced directives, sharing "bad news," personal relationship and family issues, and end-of-life concerns. Other challenges include issues associated with provider–older adult cultural differences, and numerous physiological changes common to the aging process that can affect communication.

- Informed consent agreements are written documents designed to help govern patient–provider interactions. The purpose of an informed consent agreement is to provide enough information for the patient so that he or she can make reasoned decisions about the course of treatment.

- Cultural factors and language differences can present significant challenges to securing informed consent. Another significant challenge to entering into an informed consent agreement is the use of professional jargon.

- The cornerstone of ethical service delivery, especially health care services, is the obligation to maintain patient confidentiality. Preserving and protecting patient confidentiality is central to the patient–provider relationship.

- An advance health care directive is a written document that describes a person's preferences as to which life-sustaining medical interventions he or she desires or does not desire should these interventions become necessary in the future due to a medical emergency or illness and should the individual be unable or unwilling to communicate his or her preferences at that time.

- Culturally diverse older adults may differ on issues such as the meaning of illness, the decision-making process, or concerns related to authority, respect, and control.

- The provider should be aware of his or her own tendency toward *ethnocentrism*. Ethnocentrism is a belief in the superiority of one's culture or ethnic group. Keep the older adult the focus of attention, not any perceived cultural differences.
- Providers who work within a particular cultural community different from their own would greatly benefit from seeking further information, education, and experience specific to that culture.
- Consider using a cultural brokering service or interpreter able to interpret the client's language and specific cultural nuances, as well as the health care cultures terminology.
- Age-related hearing loss can affect the ability to communicate.
- Generally speaking, age-related hearing loss has a greater impact on the ability to hear higher pitched sounds than lower pitched ones. This may make it more difficult to distinguish between certain consonants.
- Men tend to experience loss of high frequencies more than women.
- Teach-back techniques are helpful to confirm understanding of information received. They involve asking the older adult to explain—in his or her own words—what he or she has been told.
- Aphasia results from brain damage—most commonly the result of a stroke or head trauma. Aphasia does not affect intelligence, but it does impede the capacity to communicate—most notably the person's ability to speak and understand others.
- Many age-related changes that lead to cognitive impairment are associated with a decline in working memory.
- *Dementia* refers to conditions that result in deterioration of memory and cognitive processes that reduce an individual's ability to successfully perform the activities of daily living.
- Dementia can affect memory, speech, and communication. There is often difficulty with word finding, termed *anomia*. People with dementia may use nonsensical words. Focus and concentration are frequently and severely compromised. Mental wandering is common.
- The older adult with dementia may talk about unrelated topics. He or she may seem to mix past, present, and future.
- Older adults with Alzheimer's disease and other forms of dementia can pose considerable communication challenges.
- Even in late-stage dementia, the individual may understand more than is apparent and still benefit from the provider's caring, compassionate communication.

- The cognitively challenged older adult needs to be seen, heard, and treated as a unique and valued individual.
- Treat everything the older adult says as an attempt to share something important.
- Treat each person with respect and as a unique individual.
- Avoid the tendency to pre-judge. Avoid elderspeak.
- Frame communication according to the guidelines offered by the ten C's.
- The single most important fact for a provider to remember when interacting with culturally diverse older adults, or when discussing sensitive issues, or when communicating with those suffering from hearing loss, aphasia, or dementia, is that each individual is unique and wants to feel heard and valued.

## Provider Self-Test and/or Suggestions for Instructors

**Describe:** Some of the challenges faced when discussing emotionally laden topics with an older adult.

**Explain:** The purpose of informed consent and advanced directives.

**Discuss:** How cultural differences can impede accurate communication. Describe some of the ways to reduce possible misunderstanding.

**Explain:** The concept of *ethnocentrism*, and describe how it can hinder person-centered communication.

**Discuss:** The effects of age-related hearing loss on an older adult's ability to hear higher pitched sounds. Give an example of how knowledge of these effects could be used to enhance the communication process.

**Explain:** The teach-back technique. Provide an example of how a provider could use this method to check for accurate understanding.

**List:** Some of the potential risks to the older adult, the provider, and to society at large of the misunderstanding of health care–related information.

**List:** At least six of the ways a provider could enhance the communication process when interacting with an older adult suffering from age-related hearing loss.

**Discuss:** The effects of aphasia on an older adult's ability to speak and understand another person's language.

**Describe:** Some of the common symptoms of aphasia, and list at least six ways a provider could enhance the communication process when interacting with an older adult suffering from aphasia.

**Discuss:** Several of the common symptoms of Alzheimer's disease, and then describe its impact on an older adult's memory, behavior, speech, and thinking.

**Identify:** At least nine ways a provider can enhance the communication process when speaking with an older adult suffering from Alzheimer's.

## WEB RESOURCES

Alzheimer's Association
  http://www.alz.org
The American Speech-Language-Hearing Association
  www.asha.org
Hearing Loss Association of America
  www.hearingloss.org
National Aphasia Association
  http://www.aphasia.org/
National Council on Aging
  ncoa.org/HearingLoss
National Institute on Deafness and Other Communication Disorders
  http://www.nidcd.nih.gov/Pages/default.aspx

## REFERENCES

Alzheimer's Association. (2014). Alzheimer's disease facts and figures. *Alzheimer's & Dementia*, *10*(2), 1–75.
American Speech-Language-Hearing Association. (2012). www.asha.org.
Beers, M. H. (Ed.). (2004). *The Merck manual of health and aging*. New York, NY: Ballantine Books.
Drench, M. E., Noonan, A. C., Sharby, N., & Ventura, S. H. (2012). *Psychosocial aspects of health care*. Upper Straddle River, NJ: Pearson Education.
Ekerdt, D. J. (Ed.). (2002). *Encyclopedia of aging*. New York, NY: Thomson Gale.
Fremgen, B. (2006). *Medical law and ethics*. Upper Saddle River: Prentice Hall.
Harwood, J., Leibowitz, K., Lin, M., Morrow, D. G., Rucker, N. L., & Savundranayagam, M.Y. (2012). *Communicating with older adults: An evidence-based review of what really works*. Washington, DC: Gerontological Society of America.
Hummert, M. L., Wieman, J. M., & Nussbaum, J. F. (1994). *Interpersonal communication in older adulthood*. Thousand Oaks, CA: Sage Publications.
Jecker, N., Jonsen, A., & Pearlman, R. (1997). *Bioethics: An introduction to the history, methods, and practice*. Boston: Jones and Bartlett Publishers.
Jonsen, A., Siegler, M., & Winsdale, W. (2002). *Clinical ethics*. New York: McGraw-Hill.
Kemp, E. C., Floyd, M. R., McCord-Duncan, E., & Lang, F. (2008). Patients prefer the method of "tell back-collaborative inquiry" to assess understanding of medical information. *Journal of the American Board of Family Medicine, 21*(1), 24–30.
Kukla, R. (2009). Communicating consent. *Hasting Center Report, 39*(3), 45–47.
Mayo clinic. (2014), http://www.mayoclinic.org/diseases-conditions/alzheimers-disease/basics/definition/con-20023871.
National Institute on Deafness and Other Communication Disorders. (2014). http://www.nidcd.nih.gov/Pages/default.aspx.
Nussbaum, J. F., Pecchioni, L. L., Robinson, J. D., & Thompson, T. L. (2000). *Communication and aging*. Mahwah, NJ: Lawrence Erlbaum Associates.
Pautex, S., Herrman, F., & Zulian, G. (2008). Role of advance directives in palliative care units: a prospective study. *Palliative Medicine, 22*, 835–841.

Purtilo, R., & Haddad, A. (2002). *Health professional and patient interaction.* New York: W.B. Saunders Company.

Robnett, R. H., & Chop, W. C. (2010). *Gerontology for the health care professional.* Sudbury, MA: Jones and Bartlett Publishers.

Rogers, W. (2006). Pressures on confidentiality. *The Lancet, 367*(18), 554–555.

Rosner, F. (2006). Medical confidentiality and patient privacy: the Jewish perspective. *Cancer Investigation, 24*(1), 113–115.

Salimbene, S. (2000). *What language does your patient hurt in: A practical guide to culturally competent patient care.* St. Paul, MN: Paradigm Publishing.

Tamparo, C., & Lindh, W. (2008). *Therapeutic communications for health care.* Clifton Park: Delmar Learning.

Touhy, T. A., & Jett, K. F. (2011). *Ebersole & Hess' toward healthy aging: Human needs and nursing response.* St. Louis, MO: Elsevier, Mosby.

Wallhagen, M. I. (2010). The stigma of hearing loss. *Gerontologist, 50*(1), 66–75.

Waring, A. (2012). *The heart of care.* London. England: Souvenir Press.

World Health Organization. (2015). www.who.int/mediacentre/factsheets/fs300/en/.

Yang, J., & Kombarakaran, F. (2006). A practitioner's response to the new health privacy regulations. *Health and Social Work, 31*(2), 129–136.

CHAPTER 7

# Person-Centered Communication and Stress: The Eighth C—Calmness

*Every stress leaves an indelible scar, and the organism pays for its survival after a stressful situation by becoming a little older.*

**Hans Selye**

**Core Question:** How can the person-centered communication approach help lower frustration and stress for both the provider and older adult?

**Keywords:** Allostasis; Allostatic overload; Homeostasis; Professional burnout; Relaxation response; Resilience; Stress; Stress management; Stress response; Stressors.

## INTRODUCTION: THE STRESS OF COMMUNICATION

There are numerous obstacles to effective communication. Chapter 4 explored common barriers that can undermine the provider–older adult relationship and impede interpersonal communication. Chapter 5 discussed three age-related changes that can affect the communication process—hearing loss, aphasia, and cognitive impairments.

There are also several traits that encourage effective communication. One example is the practice of the first seven C's described in Chapter 4—caring, compassionate, courteous, clear, concise, congruent, and complete.

Because poor quality interpersonal communication can be a major source of stress for providers, older adults, and aging services-related organizations, this chapter introduces the eighth *C—calmness*. It includes detailed suggestions about how to develop a stress management plan of care—both for individual providers and employing organizations that ultimately results in better quality service.

## POOR COMMUNICATION AND STRESS

Providing services to older adults can be rewarding, yet demanding, frustrating, and stressful (Hart, 2010; Hulbert & Morrison, 2006; Tamparao & Lindh, 2008). A provider's communication ability often suffers under the effects of excess stress. For example, a study of medical residents found that those exposed to high levels of stress were at risk for decreased empathic response to patients, compromising the quality of interpersonal communication (Passalacqua & Segrin, 2012).

Health care-related communication can be stressful for both providers and older adults. A study of inexperienced physicians revealed that they experienced high stress levels when required to share "bad news" with a patient (Hulsman et al., 2010).

A USA Today story (Eisler, 2014) reported that data from a United States Substance Abuse and Mental Health Services Administration study conducted in 2007 revealed that approximately 103,000 health care providers each year were self-medicating and/or abusing illicit drugs. It is possible that some of this self-medicating could be stress-related.

A growing body of evidence suggests that the stress inherent to working within the aging services network, negatively impacts providers (Gelsema, van der Doef, Maes, Akerboom, & Verhoeve, 2005; Shapiro, Astin, Scott, Bishop, & Cordova, 2005). Working under increased demands for efficiency and cost effectiveness, providers face the challenge of balancing the business side of their work with the importance of their patient relationships. At the same time, consumers consistently rank the relationship with their provider as high in priority (Hart, 2010).

For the provider, chronic overexposure to stress may lead to increased difficulty adhering to the seven C's of person-centered communication, interpersonal conflicts, reduced morale, increased absenteeism and health risks, and professional burnout. For the employer, the negative impact of stressful communications can lead to problems with staff relations, reduced quality of services, increased client dissatisfaction, problems with staff retention, and increased expenses related to employee turnover. For the older adult, excessive stress can result in increased interpersonal conflict, increased dissatisfaction with provider services, poorer therapeutic outcomes, and increased health risks.

Occasionally, when a provider and older adult interact, misunderstandings occur, feelings are hurt, and frustration and stress are the result. This is especially true when discussing difficult or sensitive issues such as advanced directives or when providers experience uncertainty stemming from interacting with older adults from cultural backgrounds differing from their own. By themselves, many of these conversationally induced stressors could be viewed as minor; however, evidence suggests these relatively insignificant daily stressors can have a cumulative effect over time with negative consequences for one's physical and psychological well-being (Adwin, Jeong, Igarashi, & Spiro, 2014; Schilling & Dichl, 2014).

## THE BODY'S STRESS RESPONSE

The body's stress-response system is normally self-regulating. It is active only when necessary and inactive when no longer required (Mayo Clinic Staff, 2014).

At the appropriate stress load for any specific individual, the biochemical processes that make up the stress response can facilitate normal growth, healthy development, and wellness. But when the level of demand begins to exceed the body's capacity to adapt, the processes associated with the body's stress-response system may instead trigger pathological changes. The chronic activation of the stress-response system may place the individual at increased risk for a number of health-related problems. This is significant for both the provider's quality of service and for the effect of a lower stress interaction on the patient.

### Author's Personal Comment

As a medical social worker formerly serving in a hospice care setting, I agree that providing end-of-life care for those diagnosed with a terminal illness is often a rewarding and meaningful experience. Yet, the nature of this work exposes the provider to a variety of occupational stressors that place him or her at risk for experiencing stress, burnout, and compassion fatigue.

Working in this setting, I was able to interact with a multidisciplinary team of professionals serving a multicultural population of patients. I learned that many of the stressors I imagined were unique to the profession of social work, were also commonly experienced by physicians, nurses, nurses aids, psychologists, occupational therapists, physical therapists, speech therapists, pharmacists, case managers, bath aides, medicine aids, assisted living directors and staff, and skilled care nursing facility staff. The specific profession and service setting may have varied, but the stress of providing quality care to the older adult remained similar.

## THE EXPERIENCE OF STRESS: FIGHT-OR-FLIGHT OR TEND-AND-BEFRIEND

Stress is an integral part of the various facets of the aging services network, especially the health care system. Similar to background noise, it is so widespread that it is often taken for granted.

For the provider, stress is commonly experienced as a felt sense of urgency and crisis—feelings of being overwhelmed and unbalanced. In men, the stress response is commonly known as the fight-or-flight response. In women—under conditions of non-life-threatening stress—it is also referred to as the tend-and-befriend response (McEwen, 2005). *Tending* is nurturing behavior designed to relieve distress. *Befriending* refers to seeking and maintaining social connections (Sapolsky, 2004, p. 17).

When the stress response is triggered, approximately 1400 biochemicals are released to prepare the body to protect itself from dangerous and potentially life-threatening situations (Childre & Rozman, 2005). The survival response is also triggered by situations that are clearly not life-threatening. This is problematic. These stress-triggering situations could be anything from the provider's daily commute in slow-moving traffic, a meeting with a supervisor, being on the receiving end of an unwanted telephone call, or an interaction with a difficult older adult.

Direct-services providers are routinely exposed to a variety of common occupational stressors. Repeated exposure places them at increased risk for developing some or all of the signs and symptoms of the stress reaction. These symptoms include rapid breathing or breathlessness; rapid heart rate and/or skipped heart beats; headaches; an increase of general body aches and pains; sleep difficulties; extreme tiredness; dizziness; anxiety and depression; impatience, anger, and irritability; changes in appetite or digestion; an increase in muscle tension; changes in libido; decreased ability to concentrate; increased difficulty in making decisions; and mental confusion. Many of these symptoms can interfere with optimal communication.

To summarize, stress responses can be caused by psychological factors, including loss of social support and outlets for frustration, a perception (or worldview) of things worsening, and under some circumstances, a loss of control and of predictability (Sapolsky, 2004). This chapter argues that a person-centered, respect-based approach to communicating with older adults not only enhances satisfactory communication but also helps to lower frustration and stress. It focuses on how providers can better manage the stress often experienced and reduce its negative impact on the quality of interpersonal communication.

## DEFINITIONS OF STRESS

Hans Selye (1907–1983)—the Canadian researcher and acknowledged father of modern stress research—defined stress as "the nonspecific response of the body to any demand for change" (Childre & Rozman, 2005). The stress response is the body's reaction to that challenge or demand (Lovallo, 2005). In this view, a stressor or demand occurs that disturbs an individual's balance or homeostasis. As a result of this disturbance, the body initiates what Selye termed the *general adaptive syndrome*—the stress response—in order to reestablish homeostasis.

Thomas (1997) described stress as the result produced when a structure, system, or organism is acted on by forces that disrupt equilibrium or produce strain. These disrupting factors are referred to as stressors.

## THE STRESS RESPONSE

Between 2000 and 2010, research into the stress response has generated many fresh concepts and new terminology. Building on biomedical knowledge, the concept of stress has evolved from the original ideas proposed by Selye. The concepts of *allostasis, allostatic state*, and *allostatic overload* are now receiving much attention.

Allostasis is an extension of the concept of homeostasis. It refers to the adaptation processes of the body to stress that help maintain homeostasis— to maintain stability in the face of change. The term *allostasis* refers to the systems of the body that aid with adaptation to a stressor (McEwen, 2005).

After a taxing exposure to stress, the body's efforts to reestablish homeostasis from allostatic overload can result. Allostatic overload refers to the cumulative effect of an allostatic state (McEwen, 2005). *Allostatic states* refer to the sustained activity levels of the body's primary mediators triggered by stressors. Allostatic states can tax the body's regulatory systems and by themselves produce stress. Findings from several studies suggest that higher allostatic load is associated with negative health outcomes (Logan & Barksdale, 2008). Viewed from within this expanded perspective, a stressor can be defined as anything that disturbs allostatic balance, and the stress response is the body's attempt to reestablish allostasis. Why is this important? Too much stress can negatively affect the health of a provider and the service he or she provides.

## RESILIENCE

A relatively fresh and important concept in the study of stress is *resilience*. Wu et al. (2013) define resilience as "the ability to adapt successfully in the face of stress and adversity" (p. 1). Resilience represents successful allostasis (Logan & Barksdale, 2008).

Resilience occurs when an individual experiences stressors and is able to successfully cope with them in a constructive manner. The trait of resilience is correlated with improved mental health and lower mortality rates (Gooding, Hurst, Johnson, & Tarrier, 2012). Healthier providers who have a positive attitude help create a healthier environment that is more positively received by the patient.

## DO NO HARM REVISITED

Providers are guided by the principle of non-maleficence—*do no harm*—as discussed in Chapter 2. Based on a large body of literature describing the negative effects of stress, an argument could be made that a provider has an ethical responsibility to structure interactions in ways that minimize exposure to the common triggers of the stress response. This is important because various age-related physiological changes in the older adult lower the individual's ability to adapt to stress (Ekerdt, 2002). This means that older adults—generally more vulnerable than their younger counterparts—are at increased risk for illness and injury including the damaging effects of stress. Example: During the winter when a grocery store parking lot might be icy, an 80-year-old woman or man who slips and falls is more likely to suffer a broken hip than is a teenager.

Exposure to stress can be viewed in a similar manner. All things being equal, the same stress load will probably have a greater impact on the older adult than the teenager.

## PROVIDER STRESS

The prevention and management of workplace stress is critically important to maintaining provider well-being and performance, for improving organizational efficiency, and enhancing success (Giga, Cooper, & Faragher, 2003, p. 294). This information is especially directed to frontline service providers who need to reduce and manage stress and also to organizational administrators who want to take steps to reduce staff burnout and increase employee retention.

This chapter advocates for the implementation of individual, provider, and agency-wide stress-reduction plans. Some of the most common workplace stressors are described. Many recommendations are offered for modifying these stressors to help mitigate their undesirable impact.

## COMMUNITY LIVING, STRESS, AND THE OLDER ADULT

More than 735,000 older adults live in assisted living facilities (National Center for Assisted Living, 2010). Another 1.4 million older adults live in nursing homes (Centers for Disease Control and Prevention, 2013). The experience of community-based living is often stressful, and (as explained in Chapter 5) ageist attitudes and exposure to elderspeak can be extremely stressful and affect the older adult's ability to communicate effectively with providers. As Wykle, Kahana, and Kowal (1992) summed up, "The need to understand the impact of personnel stress on residents cannot be overstated" (p. 198).

The message is clear: Residing in residential care facilities is often a stressful experience for the older adult. Person-centered supportive communication can serve as a buffer to help mitigate the harmful effects of stress.

## STRESSORS

A stressor is a challenge or a demand. For the provider, stressors are often described as "all the things that make you feel as if there is too much to do and not enough time to do it in" (comment by an anonymous provider). Stressors can be understood as any disrupting influence that leads an individual to feeling unbalanced or overwhelmed.

Freeman and Lawlis (2001) describe the stress reaction as an adaptive physiological response that occurs when the emotions of anger, fear, or rage are expressed. These emotions are often accompanied by increased adrenaline, elevated blood pressure and blood sugar, and accelerated heart rate. These physiological responses occur as a result of the activation of the sympathetic division of the autonomic nervous system. This occurs via the two pathways of the stress response—the hypothalamic–pituitary–adrenal axis and sympathetic–adrenal–medullary axis (Freeman & Lawlis, 2001). The body's capacity for these adaptive responses are important survival mechanisms, yet if unduly prolonged can lead to dysfunction and dysregulation.

## COMMON OCCUPATIONAL STRESSORS

Stressors can originate from both external and internal sources. Based on the author's professional experience, observations, and discussions with other providers, common occupational stressors include (but are not limited to) the following:

*Environmental occupational stressors:* These are the demands and pressures made on the provider from working in a confined noisy space (multiple phones ringing, many people talking, etc.), artificial lighting, poor ventilation, variable interior temperature, commuting and parking problems, and exposure to extremes of weather.

*Social and/organizational occupational stressors:* These are service coverage pressures and demands as a result of short staffing patterns; pressure to increase patient census or customer base; time pressures associated with unpredictable or changing schedules; required attendance at long staff meetings; adjustments to ever-changing service regulations and eligibility issues; completion of complex, mandated, and often duplicative service documentation; work interruptions and unplanned interactions with colleagues; occasional criticism and/or complaints from patients, customers, colleagues, supervisors and administrators; completing professional continuing education; exposure to patient, customer, and/or family anger, fear, guilt, hopelessness, desperation, suffering, and grief; exposure to patient, customer, and/or family interpersonal conflicts; and overexposure to news coverage of local and global disasters and tragedies.

*Physiological sources of occupational stressors:* These include demands made as a result of personal or family illness or accident; major life events such as giving birth or losing a loved one; lifestyle-related factors such as ingesting too much caffeine, dehydration, poor diet, substance abuse, disturbed or inadequate sleep; and exposure to contagious diseases such as colds and flu.

*Internal sources of occupational stressors:* These are the demands and pressures generated by critical self-talk, pessimistic mental imagery, overly perfectionist and judgmental thoughts, occasional feelings of personal inadequacy due to an inability to control patient's pain or help resolve other significant symptoms or problems of the older adult, and struggles with personal and professional boundaries.

Repeated exposure to occupational stressors such as those listed can place the provider at increased risk for experiencing a stress reaction and—in more extreme cases—professional burnout.

## PROFESSIONAL BURNOUT

Burnout is characterized by physical and emotional exhaustion and possibly physical illness. According to the Centers for Disease Control and Prevention (2008), a significant correlation exists between exposure to occupational stressors and the onset of various physical, emotional, and mental health problems—all of which can affect quality of life, provider productivity, quality of interpersonal communication, and may lead to professional burnout.

Keidel (2002) views burnout as a syndrome that includes physical exhaustion, a negative job attitude and negative self-concept, and a general loss of concern for patients or clients. The provider who is experiencing burnout may feel more tired than usual and low in personal energy. She or he may have trouble arriving at work on time, may require longer and more frequent breaks, may leave work early, call in sick more often, and make more mistakes while on the job.

Payne (2001) characterizes burnout as an extreme strain reaction. This extreme strain may lead to chronic tiredness. Chronic tiredness, combined with feelings of being overwhelmed, may lead to increased expression of impatience and irritability.

Professional burnout can negatively impact the communication process and the relations with clients or customers and colleagues, as well as personal relationships. Impatience, irritability, and reduced tolerance for ambiguity can negatively impact team communication, cooperation, and reduce the overall quality of service delivery. The high cost of professional burnout can exact a toll not just from the provider but also from his/her colleagues, the employing organization, and most importantly from the older adults served.

## EFFECTS OF STAFF BURNOUT ON QUALITY OF SERVICES

The primary goal of an aging services-related organization is to provide quality service to the older adults served. Toward this end, the frontline staff—physicians, pharmacists, nurses, imaging technicians, and aides; speech, physical, occupational, and recreational therapists; chaplains, psychologists, counselors, social workers, case managers, and receptionists—shoulder the main responsibility for communicating and modeling the essence of the organization's philosophy. Living up to this responsibility, especially when working with the public, can present a challenge. Stressed out, burned out, impatient, irritable providers and staff can find it difficult or even impossible to personify the spirit of the service organization.

The quality of the relationships established among providers, staff, and the older adults served is critical to the mission and success of the service organization. Because of the importance of this professional relationship, it would seem obvious that the health and well-being of the professionals and other frontline workers is essential, both for the delivery of exceptional service and the continued success of the organization.

## STRESS AND THE PROVIDER'S PERSONAL PLAN OF CARE

Health care facilities, as well as many other types of aging services organizations, typically require that each older adult served has an individualized, written service plan or plan of care. Depending on the type of service offered, this plan of care includes goals and interventions selected to address the physical, emotional, social, financial, residential, mental, and/or spiritual concerns of the older adult. The plan of care is not a fixed, static document. It is an evolving, dynamic document—dated, updated, and reviewed at regular intervals by the provider in collaboration with the older adult.

This chapter encourages providers to develop their own personal plan of care with goals and interventions selected to address the increased risks associated with frequent exposure to occupational stressors. The SMART goal-setting method explained in Chapter 2 should prove helpful in developing a personal plan.

This chapter also encourages involved administrators and program managers to draft and implement an overall organizational plan of care. In developing the organizational plan of care, administrators could create a plan designed to provide staff with the time, training, tools, and encouragement to create their own individualized plans.

The creation of a personal stress reduction care plan for each provider could help increase awareness of the impact that repeated exposures to various occupational stressors could have on personal health and professional well-being. It could also provide interventional suggestions designed to improve coping skills and reduce stress—all of which contributes to enhanced quality of service delivery.

## THE KEY ROLE OF ORGANIZATION ADMINISTRATION

Organization administrators could play a key role in preventing or helping to reducing provider stress. They could also play an important role in preventing professional burnout through the elimination, reduction, or control of the sources of occupational stressors previously described.

Based on the author's personal observations, experience, and conversations with other professionals, the following sections offer recommendations that administration might consider to help address common occupational stressors.

## Recommendations for Environmental Occupational Stressors

1. Arrange the work environment to invite relaxed efficiency, comfort, and teamwork with adequate space, lighting, temperature, and where needed, sound-muffling separator panels. Where possible, allow each staff person maximum control over his or her own work space.
2. Encourage staff to keep noise levels appropriate to the task and setting.
3. Try to ensure staff have ample time for commuting and adequate parking spaces.
4. Create job descriptions based on actual in-the-field work models that focus on the tasks and time required for providers to fulfill them.

## Recommendations for Addressing Social and Organizational Occupational Stressors

1. If possible, staff providing direct patient care in the field could be given a specific territory so commuting times are more predictable.
2. The maximum number of patients or clients that can be assigned to any one provider should be clearly defined and communicated. Ceilings on caseloads should be respected. When patient or client census begins to regularly exceed this limit, additional on-call or permanent employees should be added as quickly as possible.
3. Provide predictable work schedules to staff. Allow staff the maximum control possible over their day-to-day schedules.
4. If possible, discourage early morning staff meetings to reduce provider exposure to rush-hour traffic and the accompanying stress. Beginning a work day under this type of stress can be counterproductive.
5. Establish a panel of direct-care and records staff to explore ways of simplifying documentation. The task of this panel might be to review all required organizational documentation with an eye toward eliminating nonrequired charting and duplication.
6. Staff in-service education could provide additional training in stress reduction, use of constructive mental imagery, time management, workplace efficiency, and aspects of certain communication skills. Conducting scenario-based communication trainings using simulated patients could prove helpful. Making use of simulated patients, clients, or residents to rehearse common communication challenges could enhance provider–older adult interactions (Wakefield, Cooke, & Boggis, 2003).

## Recommendations for Addressing Physiological Occupational Stressors

1. When possible, provide a generous amount of paid personal leave. Encourage staff to take personal leave or "wellness" days instead of allowing them to accumulate.
2. If possible, provide employer-paid wellness and lifestyle counseling. Offer wellness and fitness-based incentives (group discounts for health club memberships).

## Recommendations for Addressing Internal Stressors

1. Provide in-service education on topics such as how to develop personal and professional SMART goals, setting and adhering to professional boundaries, and integrating mindfulness into the workplace.
2. Provide individual and/or group training in the use of physical relaxation techniques, the use of stress-reducing mental imagery (explained in Chapter 8), and in methods for increasing heart-rhythm coherence (described in Chapter 9).

Adopting these recommendations could help encourage provider self-care—a trait strongly associated with enhanced wellness, professional productivity, and improved patient or customer outcomes.

## STRESS PLAN OF CARE FOR THE PROVIDER

Some degree of stress is probably healthy, motivating, and necessary for on-the-job work productivity. However, when stress occurs at levels the professional cannot process and dissipate, pathological changes may result as previously described.

Stress management for the frontline provider involves learning how to reduce exposure to stressors when possible and to counteract the potential negative effects of stress after it is triggered. It involves the application of specific skills of self-regulation, such as learning to evoke a sense of calmness, relaxation, and feeling at ease—skills that support the person-centered approach to communication.

## DEFUSING STRESS: ELICITING THE RELAXATION RESPONSE

Substantial evidence exists to show that chronic stress has a deleterious effect on physical health (Benson & Casey, 2013). Eliciting the relaxation response—a sense of calmness (the eighth C) and feeling at ease—on a regular basis can act as an antidote.

The term *relaxation response* was coined by Dr. Herbert Benson, founder of Harvard's Mind/Body Medical Institute. Essentially, the relaxation response is the opposite reaction to the fight-or-flight response. It is a deep sense of physical relaxation and mental calm. There are many ways to trigger the relaxation response. Here is an adaptation of Dr. Benson's (2000) original method:

- Sit in a comfortable position, and close your eyes.
- Settle in, and physically relax deeply from head to toe.
- Breathe through your nose, easily and naturally. As you inhale, think the word "calm" or "one." As you exhale, think the word "calm" or "one."
- When distracting thoughts occur, try to ignore them and simply return to repeating "calm" or "one."
- Continue sitting and breathing for 10–20 min. Do not try to relax. Simply sit passively, and allow relaxation to occur at its own pace.

For best results, practice eliciting the relaxation response one to two times daily. Results are cumulative. By itself, eliciting the relaxation response is highly valuable in mitigating the harmful effects of stress. It is even more effective when combined with other commonly used techniques for stress management—eating a nutritious diet, getting adequate exercise and sleep, and socializing.

Many of the following suggestions were offered by the author's colleagues who gathered together for a monthly staff support group. Several of these interventions have been discussed by Freeman and Lawlis (2001). These include affirmations, positive self-talk and self-suggestions, aroma therapy, catnaps, chamomile tea, crying, cuddling, dancing, deep breathing, exercising, hot baths or showers, humming, hypnosis, improved diet and hydration, imagery (as explained in Chapter 8), laughing, listening to relaxing music, massage, meditating and mindfulness, playing with pets and children, praying, progressive muscle relaxation, recalling pleasant memories (as described in Chapters 8 and 9), singing, spending time in nature, stretching, walking, yoga, and taking more relaxing vacations.

## Exercise: The 90-second Relaxation Break

The 90-second relaxation break is an easy-to-learn method for evoking the relaxation response. Developed by the author, it was first shared with a group of 40 hospice professionals gathered together for an in-service training on stress management. It has also been offered to hundreds of community college students enrolled in a popular course taught by the author—*Therapeutic Communication for the Health Professional*.

The 90-second relaxation break can be enjoyed whenever the provider has a few minutes. Individuals have used this to help relax and counter the effects of stress while using the rest room, before starting their car on the way to and/or from work, while on a coffee or lunch break, and upon arrival at home at the end of the work day. The benefits are both immediate and accumulative. Here's how to do it.

- Take four deep and easy breaths. Let your exhalation be slightly longer than your inhalation.
- With each breath, think the word "relax" or "calm."
- After completing four breaths, vividly recall and savor a relaxing and pleasant memory for another 10–15 seconds.
- Take one more deep and easy breath. Exhale slowly, and return to your activity.

Additional versions of this exercise are described in Chapter 9, especially those designed to increase coherence.

---

Over the years, the author has worked with hundreds of older adult clients and shared many suggestions for reducing, managing, and coping with stress. Various colleagues have also shared techniques they use and recommend for helping to manage stress. Collectively, these include suggestions to: from time to time, recall your personal reasons for entering your chosen field of work.

1. Contemplate whether the initial reasons for selecting this type of work are still valid. Examine how (or if) you continue to benefit from this work and list your reasons for continuing (or leaving) this line of work.
2. Try to keep work in perspective—strive for physical, emotional, mental, and spiritual balance. Cover your bases. Make sure you are getting adequate sleep, rest and relaxation, eating sensibly, staying well-hydrated, and enjoying regular activity, exercise, and recreation.
3. Maintain close personal relationships with family, friends, and community.
4. Know your personal and professional limitations. Learn to ask for what is needed and also how and when to say "no" to yourself, your colleagues, and even your boss.
5. Set and maintain professional boundaries. Potential warning signs that boundaries between a provider and an older adult are possibly being crossed include giving a patient, client, or customer your home phone or private cell phone number; extending visits with certain individuals beyond what is required to render the needed professional services; regularly thinking about specific patients or customers after work; forming personal rather than professional relationships—especially intimate

relations; sharing inappropriate personal information; concealing from colleagues the depth or extent of the relationship with the patient or customer; and accepting or giving inappropriate gifts or favors.

6. At the end of the day, leave your work at your place of business. To assist with letting go of the day's work concerns, a daily rite of release can be helpful—something to remind yourself the day's work is done. For example, you could listen to a specially selected piece of music as you drive home; enjoy a hot shower to cleanse away daily concerns; go for a walk or engage in any enjoyable activity as soon as you arrive home; sit down, close your eyes, and imagine the concerns of the day getting smaller and smaller and moving further and further away until they disappear; and change into non-work clothes.

7. Cultivate a supportive social network where professional concerns and feelings can be shared with trusted colleagues.

8. If available, attend staff support meetings.

Providers cannot control all of the events that happen around them. They can, however, learn to exert more conscious control over how they respond to these events. This involves cultivating the habit of responding to stressors rather than reacting to them. The technique discussed next was developed to help providers further develop this skill and was first presented by this author at a professional in-service training.

## TIME OUT FOR THE PROFESSIONAL

Climbers do not expect to scale a mountain without taking many planned rest breaks. Surprisingly though, many providers think nothing of working 12 hour days without taking any real breaks. It is common knowledge that human beings have cycles of dream sleep throughout the night at roughly 90–120 min intervals. It is also well known that people have cycles of increased and decreased energy and concentration throughout the waking part of the day.

The provider is encouraged to respect these natural daily energy cycles and develop the habit of enjoying brief time outs at regular intervals throughout the day—especially when feeling low on energy. These time outs can include activities such as short power naps, meditation, daydreaming, enjoying a brief social interlude, enjoying a short walk (even down the hall), taking a refreshment break, stretching in the restroom, doing some deep breathing combined with relaxing mental imagery, or listening to music. Like the catnap, taking a time out is simply a good investment of time that pays itself back quickly in increased productivity and reduced stress.

## THE STRESS OF COMMUTING

Providers who make home visits often spend much time commuting in heavy traffic. For most, the desire to arrive punctually for work and to quickly get back home after work is strong. This can sometimes lead to overly aggressive driving, feelings of impatience and irritability, short tempers, obscene gestures, lane switching, tailgating, horn honking, and in some cases, road rage and accidents.

The following ideas, inspired by Kabat-Zinn (1990), are for those times when the professional is commuting or stuck in heavy traffic. Collectively, they could be considered as emotional CPR—short for Choose Positive Responses.

1. Drive mindfully. Be in the present moment.
2. Breathe deeply.
3. Purposefully remind yourself that other people are also stuck in traffic the same way you are. Most likely, they are not enjoying it either.
4. Listen to some preselected relaxing music, possibly something that makes you want to sing along.
5. Whenever you are stuck in heavy traffic—at least once—consciously decide to be a "Good Samaritan" and make room for another driver to merge into traffic or change lanes.
6. Upon arrival at work, sit in your car for one minute and just breathe deeply. When finished, get out of the car and walk calmly into your place of work. Smile at the first person you see.
7. At the end of the work day, do the same as above.

## THE STRESS OF DOCUMENTATION

Any provider knows that aging services work involves documentation—and plenty of it. It comes with the territory. For example, in the health care arena, every patient served requires extensive and comprehensive medical charting. With all this required documentation, it is no surprise that many providers struggle to complete documentation in a thorough and timely manner. Yet professionals also know how important this documentation is to providing quality service and getting reimbursed for it.

The following are some suggestions to help reduce the stress associated with the completion of required documentation. These suggestions were gleaned from the author's professional experience as well as ideas shared by colleagues.

1. If using paper documentation, always have an ample supply of required forms near your work area, on your desk, and in your car.
2. Whether documentation is electronic or paper, be very familiar with the forms or software used so you can complete work quickly.
3. Have a list of stock phrases routinely used that can be adapted to the person and service rendered.
4. While completing required documentation, remind yourself that this is all related to quality patient care and reimbursement.
5. Try to develop the habit of completing documentation as soon as possible after service is completed—preferably not while you are still with the older adult.
6. If you are sitting at your desk and feeling a little overwhelmed, push your chair back, stand up, and walk away. Take a stroll to the kitchen or bathroom. Get a drink of water. Briefly chat with a colleague. Take a step outside for two to four deep breaths of fresh air. Physically removing yourself from your work area for a couple minutes can help reduce tension and stress.
7. Be willing to serve on a panel consisting of both direct-care and record staff to focus on the task of simplifying documentation. The objective of this panel would be to review all required organization documentation with an eye toward eliminating nonessential and duplicative entries.

## CONCLUSION

The negative impact of stress is cumulative. Poor quality, unsatisfactory, interpersonal communication can be a major source of stress for providers and older adults. It is not unusual for a provider's communication ability to suffer under the effects of stress. The focus of this chapter was on helping providers learn to reduce stress in order to enhance the quality of interpersonal communication and improve the provider–older adult professional relationship.

In addition to the stress of interpersonal communication, the nature of aging services work also exposes the provider to numerous occupational stressors. Whether it is the stress of interpersonal communication—difficult conversations such as advanced directives, delivering "bad news," encountering multicultural challenges, commuting, working long hours, documenting professional services—or various occupational stressors, it is important for the provider to develop a personal stress-management care plan. This can help reduce the negative consequences resulting from long-term exposure to stressors by learning to purposefully evoke feelings of calmness, the eighth C.

## LIST OF MAIN POINTS FOR PREVIEW AND REVIEW

- Substantial evidence exists to show that chronic stress has a deleterious effect on physical health, which affects the provider's performance and communication.
- The nature of aging services-related work exposes the professional to a variety of occupational stressors that place him or her at risk for experiencing stress, burnout, and compassion fatigue—all of which can negatively impact physical health and emotional well-being.
- Poor quality, unsatisfactory, interpersonal communication can be a major source of stress for providers and older adults.
- An argument could be made that a provider has an ethical responsibility to structure interactions in ways that minimize exposure to common triggers of the stress response.
- Various age-related physiological changes in the older adult lower the individual's ability to adapt to stress. This means that older adults are generally more vulnerable than their younger counterparts.
- A person-centered, respect-based approach to communicating with older adults not only enhances satisfactory communication but also helps lower frustration and stress.
- Person-centered supportive communication can serve as a buffer to help mitigate the harmful effects of stress.
- Stress is the nonspecific response of the body to any demand for change called a *stressor*. The stress response is the body's reaction to the stressor.
- A stressor or demand occurs that disturbs an individual's homeostasis. As a result of this disturbance, the body initiates the stress response in order to reestablish homeostasis.
- Allostasis is an extension of the concept of homeostasis. It refers to the adaptation processes of the body to stress that help maintain homeostasis and maintain stability in the face of change.
- Allostatic overload refers to the cumulative effect of an allostatic state. Allostatic states can tax the body's regulatory systems and by themselves produce stress.
- Higher allostatic load is associated with negative health outcomes.
- A stressor can be defined as anything that disturbs allostatic balance, and the stress response is the body's attempt to reestablish allostasis.
- Relatively minor daily stressors can have a cumulative effect over time.
- Stressors can originate from both external and internal sources, which include environmental occupational stressors, social and/organizational

occupational stressors, physiological sources of occupational stressors, and internal sources of occupational stressors.

- The chronic activation of the stress–response system may place the individual at increased risk for a number of health-related problems including professional burnout.

- The high cost of professional burnout can exact a toll not just from the provider but also from his/her colleagues, the employing organization, and most importantly from the older adults served.

- In men, the stress response is commonly known as the fight-or-flight response. In women—under conditions of non-life-threatening stress—it is also referred to as the tend-and-befriend response.

- Resilience is the ability to adapt successfully in the face of stress and adversity and is correlated with improved mental health and lower mortality rates.

- This chapter encourages providers to develop their own personal plan of care with goals and interventions selected to address the increased risks associated with frequent exposure to occupational stressors. It also encourages involved administrators and program managers to draft and implement an overall organizational plan of care.

- Stress management for the frontline professional involves the application of specific skills of self-regulation, such as learning to evoke a sense of calmness, relaxation, and feeling at ease.

- Eliciting the relaxation response—a sense of calmness and feeling at ease—on a regular basis can act as an antidote to stress.

## Provider Self-Test and/or Suggestions for Instructors

**Personal reflections:** Share personal examples of communication with a provider that felt unsatisfactory and stressful. Discuss what made the interaction feel stressful.

**Define:** The terms stress, stressors, the stress response, and stress management.

**Compare and contrast:** The stress response commonly known as the *fight-or-flight response* with the *tend-and-befriend response*.

**Discuss:** The concept of *homeostasis*. Integrate into this discussion, the concepts of *allostasis, allostatic overload*, and *resilience*.

**Discuss:** The categories of occupational stressors. Then, compare and contrast external and internal sources of stressors.

**Debate and discuss:** The argument that a provider has an ethical responsibility to structure interactions in ways that minimize exposure to common triggers of the stress response.

**Explain:** The concept of *the relaxation response*, and share several methods used for evoking it.

## WEB RESOURCES

**The American Institute of Stress**
The American Institute of Stress (AIS) was founded in 1978 at the request of Dr. Hans Selye—popularly referred to as the "father" of the stress concept.
   www.Stress.org

**Mayo Clinic – Stress**
   http://www.mayoclinic.org/healthy-living/stress-management/
   basics/stress-basics/hlv-20049495

**Medline Plus – National Institute of Health**
   http://www.nlm.nih.gov/medlineplus/ency/article/001942.htm

**Cleveland Clinic - Stress**
   http://my.clevelandclinic.org/health/healthy_living/hic_Stress_Manag
   ement_and_Emotional_Health

**Journals**
International Journal of Stress Management
   www.apa.org/pubs/journals/str/

**Recommended Books**
Childre, D., & Rozman, D. (2005). *Why zebras don't get ulcers: The acclaimed guide to stress, stress-related diseases, and coping.* New Harbinger Publications. (Kindle Edition).
Sapolsky, R. M. (2004). *Transforming stress: The heartmathsolution for relieving worry, fatigue, and tension.* Henry Holt and Co. (Kindle Edition).

## REFERENCES

Adwin, C. M., Jeong, Y., Igarashi, H., & Spiro, A. (2014). Do hassles and uplifts change with age? Longitudinal findings from the VA normative aging study. *Psychology and Aging,* 29(1), 57–71.
Benson, H. (2000). *The relaxation response.* New York, NY: Harper Collins.
Benson, H., & Casey, A. (Eds.). (2013). *Stress management approaches for preventing and reducing stress.* Boston, MA: Harvard Health Publications.
Centers for Disease Control and Prevention. (2008). *Exposure to stress: Occupational hazards in hospitals.* National Institute for Occupational Safety and Health. http://www.cdc.gov/niosh/.
Centers for Disease Control and Prevention. (2013). http://www.cdc.gov/nchs/fastats/nursing-home-care-htm.
Childre, D., & Rozman, D. (2005). *Transforming stress: The heartmath solution for relieving worry, fatigue, and tension.* New Harbinger Publications(Kindle Edition).
Eisler, P. (2014). Doctors, medical staff on drugs put patients at risk. *USA Today,* April 16, 2014, p. A.1.
Ekerdt, D. J. (Ed.). (2002). *Encyclopedia of aging, volume 4: Q-z.* Farmington Hills, MI: The Gale Group.

Freeman, L. W., & Lawlis, G. F. (2001). *Mosby's complementary and alternative medicine: A research-based approach*. St. Louis: Mosby.

Gelsema, T. I., van der Doef, M., Maes, S., Akerboom, S., & Verhoeve (2005). Job stress in the nursing profession: the influence of organizational and environmental conditions and job characteristics. *International Journal of Stress Management, 12*(3), 222–240.

Giga, S. I., Cooper, C. L., & Faragher, B. (2003). The development of a framework for a comprehensive approach to stress management interventions at work. *International Journal of Stress Management Copyright, 10*(4), 280–296.

Gooding, P. A., Hurst, A., Johnson, J., & Tarrier, N. (2012). Psychological resilience in young and older adults. *International Journal of Geriatric Psychiatry, 27*, 262–270.

Hart, J. (2010). Teaching humanism in medical training. *Alternative and Complementary Therapies, 17*(1), 9–13.

Hulbert, N. J., & Morrison, V. L. (2006). A preliminary study into stress in palliative care: optimism, self-efficacy and social support. *Psychology, Health, and Medicine, 11*(2), 246–254.

Hulsman, R. L., Pranger, S., Koot, S., Fabriek, M., Karemaker, J. M., & Smets, E. M. A. (2010). How stressful is doctor-patient communication? Physiological and psychological stress of medical students in simulated history taking and bad-news consultations. *International Journal of Psychophysiology, 77*(1), 26–34.

Keidel, G. C. (2002). Burnout and compassion fatigue among hospice caregivers. *American Journal of Hospice and Palliative Medicine, 19*(3), 200–205.

Kabat-Zinn, J. (1990). *Full catastrophe living: Using the wisdom of your body and mind to face stress, pain, and illness*. New York, NY: Bantam Dell.

Logan, J. G., & Barksdale, D. J. (2008). Allostasis and allostatic load: expanding the discourse on stress and cardiovasculular disease. *Journal of Clinical Nursing, 17*(7B), 201–208.

Lovallo, W. R. (2005). *Stress and health biological and psychological interactions*. Thousand Oaks: Sage Publications.

Mayo Clinic Staff. (2014). http://www.mayoclinic.org/healthy-living/stress-management/basics/stress-basics/hlv-20049495.

McEwen, B. S. (2005). Stressed or stressed out: what is the difference? *Journal Psychiatry Neuroscience, 30*(5), 315–318.

National Center for Assisted Living. (2010). http://www.ahcancal.org/ncal/Pages/index.aspx.

Passalacqua, S. A., & Segrin, C. (2012). The effect of resident physician stress, burnout, and empathy on patient-centered communication during the long-call shift. *Health Communication, 27*(5), 449–456.

Payne, N. (2001). Occupational stressors and coping as determinants of burnout in female hospice nurses. *Journal of Advanced Nursing, 33*(3), 396–405.

Sapolsky, R. M. (2004). *Why zebras don't get ulcers: The acclaimed guide to stress, stress-related diseases, and coping*. Henry Holt and Co. (Kindle Edition).

Schilling, O. K., & Dichl, M. (2014). Reactivity to stressor pile-up in adulthood: effects on daily negative and positive affect. *Psychology and Aging, 1*, 72–83.

Shapiro, S. L., Astin, J., Scott, R., Bishop, S. R., & Cordova, M. (2005). Mindfulness-based stress reduction for health care professionals: results from a randomized trial. *International Journal of Stress Management, 12*(2), 164–175.

Tamparao, C. D., & Lindh, W. Q. (2008). *Therapeutic communication for health care*. Clifton Park, NY: Thomson Delmar Learning.

Thomas, C. (1997). *Taber's cyclopedic medical dictionary: 18th edition*. Philadelphia, PA: F.A. Davis Company.

Wakefield, A., Cooke, S., & Boggis, C. (2003). Learning together: use of simulated patients with nursing and medical students for breaking bad news. *International journal of palliative nursing, 9*(1), 32–38.

Wu, G., Feder, A., Cohen, H., Kim, J. J., Calderon, S., Charney, D. S., et al. (2013). Understanding resilience. *Frontiers in Behavioral Neuroscience, 7*(10), 1–15.

Wykle, M. L., Kahana, E., & Kowal, J. (Eds.). (1992). *Stress & health among the elderly*. New York, NY: Springer Publishing Co.

# CHAPTER 8

# Person-Centered Communication: Mental Imagery and Imagined Interactions

*The first step to better times is to imagine them.*

**From a Chinese fortune cookie**

**Core Question:** How can mental imagery be used to improve the quality of provider/older adult interpersonal communication?

**Keywords:** Active imagery; Daydreaming; End-state imagery; Functional equivalence; Guided imagery; Imagined interactions; Mental imagery; Process-based imagery; Receptive imagery; Safe place.

## INTRODUCTION

Mental imagery plays a significant and influential role in the interpersonal communication process. When a provider and an older adult interact, both individuals are creating mental images–images that can either support or hinder the communication process (Achterberg, 1985). Although the imagery generated during these interactions usually remains outside of conscious awareness, it can still influence outcomes.

Increasing numbers of physicians, nurses, psychologists, counselors, social workers, and other aging-services related professionals recognize the value and importance of imagery. Some providers may question the necessity for exploring the use of mental imagery. This chapter argues that not only does mental imagery play a significant role in the communication process, it is also an effective tool that providers can use to help lower stress and accelerate development of the traits and skills associated with the person-centered approach to communication. These include caring, compassion, congruence, empathy, genuineness, listening, mindfulness, nontechnical plain talk, patience, rapport, reduction of ageist language, relationship building, and respect. Mental imagery can also assist providers in achieving SMART-based goals as discussed in Chapter 2 and in achieving greater coherence as explained in Chapter 9.

*Person-Centered Communication with Older Adults*
http://dx.doi.org/10.1016/B978-0-12-420132-3.00008-8

131

## EVIDENCE FOR THE EFFICACY OF IMAGERY

Guided imagery has been used in pain management for centuries (Achterberg, 1985). Research from the past 30–40 years has consistently demonstrated the benefits of imagery in pain reduction and in the promotion of health (Sheikh, 2003).

In dozens of studies, imagery has been shown to affect almost all major physiologic systems of the body—blood lipids, blood pressure, cortisol levels, gastrointestinal mobility and secretion, heart rate, immune responsiveness, metabolic rates in cells, respiration, and sexual function (Freeman & Lawlis, 2001).

During the past several decades, imagery-based techniques have been in use by individuals and in clinical settings to influence health-related outcomes. Substantial evidence also exists supporting the role of imagery in the management of anxiety, depression, hypertension, pain, preparation for medical procedures, side effects related to chemotherapy, stress, and to help reduce the length of hospital stays (Hart, 2008).

Within the behavioral medicine literature, imagery is a widely accepted approach that is viewed as highly effective. In this era when the search for "high-yield" techniques is paramount, the use of mental imagery by providers for older adults is an easy-to-learn, easy-to-apply, evidence-based approach that can help improve interpersonal communications and lower the stress of both the provider and older adult.

## LEARNING CURVES AND DEVELOPMENTAL TRAJECTORIES

The provider who wants to learn how to use mental imagery for the purposes described above will face a familiar learning curve and developmental trajectory that progresses through the three stages of motivation, knowledge, and skill building as described in Chapter 2.

The provider's acquisition and mastery of specific imagery-based skills will unfold through four phases as they move from the level of beginner (unconscious incompetence) to the level of mastery (unconscious competence). The keys to continued progress are practice, persistence, and patience.

## HISTORICAL USE OF MENTAL IMAGERY

The practice of imagery is as old as human culture (Achterberg, 1985). Before the creation of words (prior to the development of word-based languages), the human thought process most likely utilized a type of sensory-based mental language, a language of imagery (Epstein & Fedoroff, 2012; Sheikh, 2002).

The term *imagery* can sometimes be confusing because it seems to refer to the visual aspect of thought. In actuality, *imagery* refers not only to visual impressions, but to the entire sensory-based thought process that includes the senses of vision, sound, touch, smell, and taste (Bone & Ellen, 1992). Imagery is multisensory.

Within the stream of human consciousness, images are one of the main ways that thoughts are expressed (Hackman, Bennett-Levy, & Holmes, 2011). Although word-based languages are now in universal use for interpersonal communication and intrapersonal communication— communication that occurs within the individual—still relies heavily on mental imagery. On a personal level, imagery is used to recall the past, capture the present moment, and anticipate the future.

## CONTEMPORARY PROFESSIONAL APPLICATIONS OF MENTAL IMAGERY

In the medical field, guided mental imagery is employed by various medical personnel for a number of patient concerns. Examples include emergency management of bleeding, fertility and/or birthing issues, pain control, needle phobia, sleep disorders, and chemotherapy and dialysis. Mental imagery is also used to help with immune system problems, stroke rehabilitation, and with the pre-preparation and post-recovery processes associated with various medical and dental procedures.

Within the domain of psychotherapy, there is a long history involving diverse applications of mental imagery. Contemporary psychiatrists, psychologists, counselors, social workers, and hypnotherapists—representing many differing therapeutic orientations—often use imagery-based techniques when conducting therapy. This is especially true in the treatment of anxiety, depression, grief, habit control, fears and phobias, relaxation training, and stress management. A sample of psychotherapeutic orientations and/or interventions that include or emphasize use of mental imagery include Gestalt therapy, guided affect therapy, multimodal therapy, cognitive-behavioral therapy, hypnosis, biofeedback, inner advisor technique, rational emotive therapy, systematic desensitization, focusing, psychosynthesis, and neuro-linguistic programming (Shor, 1983).

Within the interdisciplinary field of sports psychology, the use of mental imagery is widely accepted as an effective method for improving athletic performance (Murphy, 2005; Tenenbaum & Eklund, 2007). Although effective, Carlstedt (2013) cautions, "The notion that visualization is some sort of panacea and that it can be used by all athletes to enhance performance and that it will work, is simplistic" (p. 351).

In the field of education, guided imagery is frequently used throughout the learning process. Research suggests that the use of imagery can facilitate gains in the acquisition of academic skills (Drake, 2003). It also plays a significant role in enhancement of creativity and in the appreciation and application of the creative arts.

Members of social and business circles often employ mental rehearsal in preparation for important meetings, sales presentations, or social interactions. Professional associations exist dedicated exclusively to the research and advocacy of mental imagery. Examples include *Imagery International* and the *International Imagery Association*. *The Journal of Mental Imagery* has been in print since 1977. For providers who desire professional-level training in the use of mental imagery, courses are available from several sources: select universities, continuing education organizations, and from the *Academy for Guided Imagery*.

## IMAGERY: SELF-DIRECTED OR GUIDED, RECEPTIVE OR ACTIVE

The process of mental imagery can be self-directed or guided by another. When the process is guided by another—for example by a therapist—it is often referred to as guided mental imagery as opposed to self-directed.

Mental imagery can be *receptive* or *active* (Achterberg, Dossey, & Kolkmeier, 1994). Receptive imagery arises automatically, spontaneously appearing from "out of the blue." Active imagery is consciously and deliberately evoked and shaped by personal desire and will.

## PROCESS IMAGERY AND END-STATE IMAGERY

There are two main types of mental imagery: *process imagery* and *end-state imagery* (Achterberg et al., 1994). Process imagery refers to the use of mental imagery to explore the step-by-step procedures of how to accomplish, achieve, assemble, build, create, or understand something. It is a sequential visualization. Using process imagery, attention is focused mainly on the steps (or procedures) rather than the outcome. Process imagery can be very helpful in learning complex movements such as multistep, medical procedures.

Example: Suppose a provider named Carl decides to improve his person-centered listening skills. Using process imagery, Carl imagines sitting down and facing his older adult client. He makes eye contact. He can hear his client talking about needs and concerns. Carl imagines himself leaning forward slightly to demonstrate he is paying attention. He observes the facial expressions of his client as he listens attentively to the content and understands it. He can hear the tone of his client's voice and feels his own head nodding to show support.

End-state imagery involves using the imagination to visualize the final goal, the completed task—the outcome of the process-based imagery. Example: Carl decides to improve his person-centered listening skills. Using end-state imagery, Carl imagines hearing his client tell him, "Carl, I really appreciate how you listen to me. Talking with you, I always feel that I've been listened to and heard." Carl feels pleased with his ability to listen.

Providers may use either process-based or end-state mental imagery. Although personal preference can be used as a guideline, some recommend using process imagery first, followed by end-state imagery (Achterberg et al., 1994). Continuing with Carl's example, Carl could begin his use of mental imagery by first using process imagery, and then complete the process by employing end-state imagery.

There may be specific tasks and contexts where each version of imagery is better suited than the other. This is probably a matter of preference, best discovered through personal experience. When the steps of a specific task are unclear or the process is unknown, end-state imagery can be used by itself.

## Clinical Case Example: Process Imagery with a Patient

During a discussion with the author, a patient described how a medical assistant had used process-based guided mental imagery to help her prepare for an endoscopic examination of the throat—a procedure she found frightening. The assistant explained to her that an endoscope is a medical device consisting of a long, thin tube that includes a light and video camera (Thomas, 1997). It is used to view and record interior images of a patient's body.

The patient was then asked to close her eyes, listen, and mentally follow along while the assistant described the procedural process. She listened carefully as the assistant explained that the procedure was necessary to help arrive at an accurate diagnosis, and it would only require a few minutes. He explained that a nasal spray would be used as a mild numbing agent. After application of the numbing agent, the assistant would leave the room, and in a few minutes, the doctor would arrive to conduct the endoscopic procedure.

The doctor would insert a thin tube into her nose. This tube has a camera built into it. The flexible tube would pass up and over a bump at the top of the nose, and as it did, she would feel momentary pressure. After a few seconds, the tube would continue down her throat. She was instructed to sit very still during this procedure, and once again, was reassured the entire process would last only a few minutes.

When the examination was complete, the doctor would gently pull the tube out as she exhaled through her mouth. There might be some mild pressure experienced as the tube passed through the nasal passageway.

## Author's Comment

The assistant did an excellent job of explaining the planned medical procedure using guided imagery to assist the patient to more accurately envision the procedure. In doing so, the assistant utilized a person-centered, respectful, nontechnical approach that helped the patient feel more informed and mentally prepared. The patient felt reassured by this explanation. She especially appreciated being told how long the procedure would require. Knowing this helped reduce her fear of the "unpredictable" and the unknown. She reported the procedure went almost exactly as the assistant had described. The formula followed by the assistant can be used by other providers. The steps used were the following:

1. Name the procedure: "We're going to do an endoscopic examination of the throat." This helps reduce the patient's fear of the unknown.
2. Explain why the procedure is necessary: "This procedure is needed because_____." This rationale gives the patient a reason to endure the procedure.
3. Explain how much time the procedure will require: "The procedure will take only a few minutes." This helps reduce the patient's fear of the unpredictable.
4. Help the individual imagine the procedural steps that will be followed by describing them in nontechnical language: "Here are the steps involved in the procedure…" Again, this helps reduce fear of the unknown, thereby reducing stress.
5. Describe what the patient will most likely experience: "Here's what you'll probably feel…" This reduces fear of the unknown and fear of the unpredictable, and helps the patient feel more confident in handling it.

## DAYDREAMS, IMAGINED INTERACTIONS, IMAGINAL COMMUNICATION

Every day people imagine or daydream about conversations with family, friends, colleagues, patients, and customers that they have already had, will have, or may never have. These are imagined interactions.

*Imagined interaction* refers to a process whereby an individual imagines himself or herself in future and/or past communicative encounters with others (Honeycutt, 2003). Social scientists have been studying imagined interactions since the mid-1980s (Honeycutt, 2010).

In this book, the concept of *imaginal communication* refers to a method for employing mental imagery or daydreaming as a tool that can be used for improving the effectiveness of communication between the provider and the older adult. The APA *College Dictionary of Psychology* (2009) defines a *daydream as* "a waking fantasy or reverie, in which, expectations, and other potentialities are played out in imagination" (VandenBos, 2009, p. 96).

Daydreaming—a type of mind-wandering—is a private, normal, and virtually universal human phenomenon that forms a significant part of an individual's daily stream of consciousness. The experience of daydreaming is so widespread that it is frequently considered as the default state of the brain that emerges when the demand for external, task-oriented attention is reduced.

Imagined interactions are similar to daydreaming in that an individual mentally contemplates having a conversation with another person (Honeycutt, 2003). Common examples include mentally replaying a conversation after an argument with another person and fantasizing about what could have been said or done differently; mentally rehearsing an upcoming interaction with a supervisor, colleague, or meeting with board members; and imagining a different approach to communicating with a challenging patient, client, customer, or resident.

One benefit of imagined interactions is they allow a provider to imagine the outcome of alternative approaches prior to or after an actual interaction (Honeycutt, 2003). Imagining conversations before or after they take place is a tool the provider can use to help develop greater communication fluency and competency and to reduce frustration and stress. Daydreaming and imagined interactions can be used for relaxation training, stress reduction, mental rehearsal of future events and interactions, and review and editing of historical events, to name a few (Singer & Switzer, 1980).

## THE SAFE PLACE: A STAGING AREA FOR MENTAL REHEARSAL

The *safe place* is accessed via vivid imagination. It serves as a mental staging area—a safe place where the provider can quietly engage in mental imagery or mental rehearsal of a person-centered communication skill or an upcoming interaction with a challenging older adult. With practice, the safe place can function as a mental cue or trigger for quickly evoking physical relaxation and mental preparedness.

The safe place is any preselected mental image (or memory) of a private location or place where the provider feels safe and at ease. It can be an actual location or place the provider has visited (or would like to visit)—such as a secluded Hawaiian beach—or it can be an imaginary location. Here's how to use the concept of the safe place:

1. Form a clear intention for mental rehearsal or daydreaming.
2. Select a personally meaningful "safe place." Imagine being in your safe place now. Vividly recall or daydream being in your safe place for about 30–60 s.
3. While in your safe place, engage in 60–90 s of mental rehearsal or day-dreaming that expresses your intention. Example: Feeling relaxed, you daydream or use end-state imagery to see/hear/feel yourself enjoying a conversation with a previously challenging older adult patient.

## USING IMAGERY AND DAYDREAMING TO IMPROVE COMMUNICATION

New attitudes, behaviors, and skills can be practiced first in imagination before being carried out in vivo. This is referred to as *covert rehearsal* in the behavioral therapy literature (Bellack & Hersen, 1985).

Using process imagery, mental rehearsal can break complex behaviors or skills into smaller chunks of information that form a chain of information so that when the steps are performed in sequence, the target behavior is achieved. Providers usually image from beginning to end (referred to as *forward chaining*), but some also prefer to image from end to beginning (referred to as *backward chaining*). Like many aspects of mental imagery, this is probably a personal preference best discovered through experience.

1. Identify the goal of imagery. Example: "I want to improve my listening skills so I can provide the best services to my client."
2. Go to your "safe place." Relax deeply. Warm up the mental engine by recalling past successes and gradually blend your thoughts into a mental rehearsal of future goals. Develop images or daydream about your concern or desire. Example: Use mental imagery to imagine yourself using excellent listening skills in an interaction with an older adult. See and hear what you would do if actually there (use process imagery). Allow your senses to experience everything as if it is actually happening. See the environment where this interaction is occurring and the person you are interacting with. The law of exercise specificity (Di Naso, 2006) applied to mental imagery would suggest there should be a strong similarity between mental training and the real-world task or skill it is supposed to improve.
3. Try switching perspectives and see and hear your display of excellent listening skills from the vantage point of the older adult. Experience

what you would be seeing and hearing if you were the older adult. Switch perspectives once again, and assume the position of an outside observer. How do you look and sound now?

**4.** End with images of the desired state (use end-state imagery). Example: See and hear the older adult commenting on what a wonderful listener you are.

## PHYSIOLOGIC MECHANISMS OF IMAGERY AND IMAGINAL INTERACTIONS

The psychophysiology of mental imagery is well documented (Freeman & Lawlis, 2001). The use of imagery can result in physiologic, biochemical, and emotional changes in the body. Imaginary experiences activate image-relevant behavioral, cognitive, neurological, and other physiological processes.

One of the keys to understanding the effectiveness of mental imagery is contained in the concept of *functional equivalence*—the idea that visual images use the same parts of the brain as visual processing (Murphy, 2005). Neuroimaging studies suggest mental imagery is "functionally equivalent" to perception because these two types of cognitive activity share similar neural pathways (Lavallee, Kremer, Moran, & Williams, 2004).

Mental practice is functionally equivalent to physical practice. Imagination affects the brain and associated physiological processes in a way that mirrors actual, external, sensory-driven experience. For example, research shows that imagining a specific social situation can have similar effects as the actual experience (Crisp, 2009). When an individual engages in mental imagery, a plethora of electrical and chemical activity results. These results can be seen by viewing electroencephalogram records of brain waves or PET scans. Example: For a music therapist who plays guitar at a local senior center, simply imagining playing the guitar can strengthen the brain's neural connections associated with that activity. The body tends to respond to imagery as it would to a genuine external experience. When mental imagery is used repeatedly to imagine completing a specific behavior or skill, the connections between the brain's neurons associated with that action are strengthened—neurons that fire together, wire together. This is a well-researched principle of learning referred to as Hebb's Law (Whitmore, 2009).

The act of worrying is an example of the psychophysiological power of imagery. When an individual focuses on thoughts of danger—which may or may not come to pass—the body becomes tense and aroused, anticipating a threat or challenge. The fight-or-flight response is activated (Rossman, 2000, p. 35).

---

### Consider This: The Story of Two Nurses

Two nurses will soon enter the room of their next patient. Both have excellent medical skills and share similar educational and experiential backgrounds. Nurse A just spent 2 min mentally replaying the insults endured from her previous visit with an irate patient. Nurse B just spent 2 min recollecting the wonderful visit she recently enjoyed with her three-year-old grandson. Despite their similarities, it is likely that each nurse will enter the room of the next patient in very different states of emotional readiness. Nurse A might have to exert more effort than nurse B in order to provide the compassionate, person-centered approach to the communication process that the patient needs.

If the next patient was you, which nurse would you want to enter your room?

**Suggested Application:** Spend 60–90 s daydreaming about how to be more patient, respectful, and person centered with older adults. It is a simple strategy for rehearsing basic, respect-based communication skills.

---

## HOW TO SCRIPT AND DIRECT MENTAL IMAGERY

The process of mental imagery is similar to the process of scripting and directing a movie—a movie of the mind. Research suggests certain factors help maximize effectiveness of imagery (Asken, Grossman, & Christensen, 2010).

General guidelines include the following: practice mental imagery with eyes closed and eyes open, use an internal and/or external viewpoint and vividly focus on what would be seen, heard, felt, and sensed—physically and emotionally. Imagine correct responses in all senses—in real time at actual speed. Try incorporating kinesthetic imagery. This means to slightly mimic actual movements, use mini–movements, and mouth the words, where appropriate.

1. What is the setting for this mental movie? A medical office, clinic, private practice, or hospital? A residential, skilled nursing care or rehabilitation facility? Home health or hospice? A pharmacy or other commercial establishment? Where does the story take place?

2. Who are the main characters in this mental movie? Are there any supporting characters? Colleagues and/or supervisors? Family members?

3. What is the main plot of this mental movie? What is the main problem or concern that the characters hope to resolve? What are they trying to accomplish or achieve? Practice using scenario-based training based on real-life interactions likely to be encountered. Mentally rehearse the traits,

attitudes, or skills required to achieve a desirable outcome. Use 60–90 s of mental imagery to improve skills, simulate interactions and response preparation, support skill maintenance, and/or analyze and modify previous interactions (Asken et al., 2010). Rerun memories of previous interactions that need "editing" to achieve a more desirable ending.

4. Decide whether this movie will be filmed in first-person—through the provider's eyes—through the eyes of the older adult, from the perspective of a third party, or a combination of all points of view.

5. How does this mental movie end? What does a successful outcome look, sound, and feel like?

## CONCLUSION

Mental imagery plays an important role in the interpersonal communication process. It is an easy-to-learn, easy-to-apply, evidence-based approach.

The use of mental imagery allows a provider to imagine the potential outcome of various approaches to an actual interaction with an older adult. Providers can use imagery to help reduce personal stress, increase personal coherence (as described in Chapter 9), develop person-centered communication skills, improve the provider/older adult relationship, and enhance the overall quality of service delivery.

## LIST OF MAIN POINTS FOR PREVIEW AND REVIEW

- Mental imagery plays a significant role in the communication process.
- Providers can use mental imagery to help develop the traits and skills associated with the person-centered approach to communication.
- Imagery is multisensory and refers not only to visual impressions but to the entire sensory-based thought process that includes the sense of vision, sound, touch, smell, and taste.
- Mental imagery can be *receptive* or *active*.
- The process of mental imagery can be self-directed or guided by another.
- The use of imagery can result in physiologic, biochemical, and emotional changes in the body. Imaginary experiences activate image-relevant behavioral, cognitive, neurological, and other physiological processes.
- One of the keys to understanding the effectiveness of mental imagery is contained in the concept of *functional equivalence*—the idea that visual images use the same parts of the brain as visual processing.

- The safe place is an imaginary staging area where mental rehearsal and daydreaming is conducted.
- Imagined interaction refers to a process whereby a provider imagines him or herself in future and/or past communicative encounters with others.
- Imagined interactions allow a provider to imagine the potential outcome of various approaches prior to or after an actual interaction.

---

**Provider Self-Test and/or Suggestions for Instructors**

**Define and discuss key concepts:** Active imagery, daydreaming, end-state imagery, functional equivalence, guided mental imagery, imagined interactions, mental imagery, mental rehearsal, process-based imagery, receptive imagery, and safe place.

**Explain:** How mental imagery influences the communication process during interactions between two individuals.

**Discuss:** How providers can use mental imagery to improve the quality of interpersonal communications with older adults.

**Compare and contrast:** Process imagery and end-state imagery.

**Discuss:** Ways that process imagery could be used to provide reassurance to a nervous patient or client.

**Explain:** How a provider could use daydreaming to help prepare for a potentially challenging interaction with an older adult, colleague, or supervisor.

**Share:** Experiences from past professional situations where the use of mental imagery might have proven helpful. Explain how mental imagery can be used to "edit" past experience to arrive at a more desirable outcome.

**Explain:** How mental imagery can be used to develop the traits and skills associated with the person-centered approach to communication.

---

## WEB RESOURCES

Academy for guided imagery
    http://acadgi.com/
Imagery international
    http://imageryinternational.org/
*Journal of Mental Imagery*
    http://www.journalofmentalimagery.com/

## REFERENCES

Achterberg, J. (1985). *Imagery and healing: Shamanism and modern medicine*. Boston, MA: Shambhala Publications.

Achterberg, J., Dossey, B., & Kolkmeier, L. (1994). *Rituals of healing: Using imagery for health and wellness*. New York: Bantam Books.

Asken, M. J., Grossman, D., & Christensen, L. W. (2010). *Warrior mindset: Mental toughness skills for a nation's peacekeepers*. Mascoutah, IL: Human Factor's Research.

Bellack, A. S., & Hersen, M. (1985). *Dictionary of behavior therapy techniques*. Elmsford, NY: Pergamon Press.

Bone, P. F., & Ellen, P. S. (1992). The generation and consequences of communication-evoked imagery. *Journal of Consumer Research, 19*, 93–104.

Carlstedt, R. A. (2013). *Evidence-based applied sport psychology: A practitioner's manual*. New York: Springer Publishing Co.

Crisp, R. J. (2009). Can imagined interactions produce positive perceptions? Reducing prejudice through simulated social contact. *American Psychologist, 64*(4), 231–240.

Di Naso, J. (2006). *The law of exercise specificity: Is your workout really going to help you in the field?*. http://www.policeone.com/health-fitness/articles/134677-The-Law-of-Exercise-Specificity-Is-your-workout-really-going-to-help-you-in-the-field/.

Drake, S. M. (2003). Guided imagery and education: theory, practice and experience. *Journal of Mental Imagery, 27*(1–2), 94–132.

Epstein, G., & Federoff, B. L. (2012). *The encyclopedia of mental imagery*. New York: ACMI Press.

Freeman, L. W., & Lawlis, F. G. (2001). *Mosby's complementary and alternative medicine: A research based approach*. St Louis, MO: Mosby.

Hackman, A., Bennett-Levy, J., & Holmes, E. A. (2011). *Oxford guide to imagery in cognitive therapy*. New York: Oxford University Press.

Hart, J. (2008). Guided imagery. *Alternative and Complementary Therapies, 14*(6), 295–299.

Honeycutt, J. M. (2003). *Imagined interactions: Daydreaming about communication*. Cresskill, NJ: Hampton Press, Inc.

Honeycutt, J. M. (Ed.). (2010). *Imagine that: Studies in imagined interactions*. Creskill, NJ: Hampton Press.

Lavallee, D., Kremer, J., Moran, A. P., & Williams, M. (2004). *Sport psychology: Contemporary themes*. New York: Palgrave Macmillan.

Murphy, S. (2005). *The sport psychology handbook*. Champaign, IL: Human Kinetics.

Rossman, M. L. (2000). *Guided imagery for self-healing: An essential resource for anyone seeking wellness*. Novato, CA: New World Library.

Sheikh, A. (Ed.). (2002). *Handbook of therapeutic imagery*. Amityville, NY: Baywood Publishing.

Sheikh, A. (Ed.). (2003). *Healing images: The role of the imagination in health*. Amityville, NY: Baywood.

Shor, J. (1983). *Psychotherapy through imagery*. New York: Thieme-Stratton, Inc.

Singer, J. L., & Switzer, E. (1980). *Mind-play: The creative uses of fantasy*. Englewood Cliffs, NJ: Prentice-Hall, Inc.

Tenenbaum, G., & Eklund, R. C. (Eds.). (2007). *Handbook of sports psychology*. Hoboken, NJ: John Wiley & Sons, Inc.

Thomas, C. L. (1997). *Taber's cylopedic medical dictionary*. Philadelphia, PA: F.A. Davis Company.

VandenBos, G. R. (Ed.). (2009). *The APA college dictionary of psychology*. Washington, DC: American Psychological Association.

Whitmor, P. G. (2009). A new mindset for a new mind: understanding new theories about how the brain works, and what it can mean for adult learning. *American Society for Training and Development: T+D*, 60–65. http://www.astd.org/.

# CHAPTER 9

# Neurocardiology of Communication: The Ninth C—Coherence

*The heart is the chief feature of a functioning mind.*

**Frank Lloyd Wright**

**Core Question:** How can a provider use findings from the field of neurocardiology to enhance the person-centered, interpersonal communication process?

**Keywords:** Cardioelectromagnetic communication; Coherence; Distant intentionality; Entrainment; Heart rate variability; Neurocardiology.

## INTRODUCTION

Chapter 4 introduced the seven *C*'s, the main characteristics associated with effective, person-centered interpersonal communication—caring, compassionate, courteous, clear, concise, congruent, and complete. Three special *C*'s were also mentioned—calmness, coherence, and connection. Chapter 7 focused on the eighth *C*, calmness. This chapter introduces the underappreciated but very important topic of neurocardiology and discusses the heart–brain partnership. How these two organs interact and the impact this interaction has on the communication process will be explored, with emphasis on the concept of *coherence*—the next of the special *C*'s.

Interpersonal communication is the exchange of meaningful information between two or more individuals using a mutually understood language (Berry, 2007). Recent research findings from the domains of psychology, parapsychology, and physics offer fresh insights and an expanded view of the communication process.

In a wide-ranging exploration, this chapter and the next focus on several related but under-discussed topics relevant to the person-centered approach to communication. Some topics are considered speculative. Others, although evidence-based, remain controversial. But all are pertinent and offer the potential to enhance the provider–older adult relationship.

*Person-Centered Communication with Older Adults*
http://dx.doi.org/10.1016/B978-0-12-420132-3.00009-X

145

This chapter introduces some of the lesser known dynamics of the interpersonal communication process—specifically the role of the heart in the process of communication. Experimental evidence suggests that the heart's electromagnetic field may be an important source of information exchange between individuals. This exchange of information is referred to as *cardioelectromagnetic communication* (McCraty, Atkinson, & Bradley, 2004; McCraty, Atkinson, Tomasino, & Bradley, 2009).

If cardioelectromagnetic communication is taking place between a provider and an older adult, this could have important implications and practical applications. For example, this research suggests that the heart signals from one person can affect another person's brain waves. When two people are within conversational range—for example, a provider and an older adult—the electromagnetic signals generated by each individual's heart can influence the other person's brain waves. Because of this reciprocal heart–brain interaction, the physical proximity between individuals may be an important factor capable of influencing the performance of each person's brain.

During a conversational interaction, the influence exerted on each individual's brain by the other person's electromagnetic field can impact the interpersonal communication process. One important type of information that is transmitted via the cardioelectromagnetic communication process is termed *coherence*—discussed in a later section.

## PATHWAYS OF CONNECTION AND COMMUNICATION

Disciplined inquiry into the pathways and mechanisms of human interconnection reveals that interpersonal communication may be a multifaceted and multidimensional phenomenon—a process that extends beyond the simple exchange of verbal and nonverbal language. For example, studies focused on distant intentionality—the effect of human intention at a distance—provide evidence that human intention can operate between individuals at a distance (Achterberg et al., 2005).

Other lines of research suggest communication can occur between two or more persons via information-rich fields of electromagnetic energy (Combs, Arcari, & Krippner, 2006). This field-based communication occurs outside of personal awareness. The next chapter explores theories of how this interaction might take place between individuals that (in theory) are energetically entangled and interconnected at the quantum level of existence (Achterberg et al., 2005; Combs et al., 2006; Laszlo, 2006; McCraty et al., 2009). This chapter and Chapter 10 offer speculations on how these models of human connection and interaction might influence the communication process and impact the provider–older adult relationship.

## NEUROCARDIOLOGY

The most immediately applicable topic introduced in this chapter is *neurocardiology* and the role it plays in the interpersonal communication process. Neurocardiology is the specialty that deals with the brain–heart connection (van der Wall, 2011).

The body of literature related to this field has seen rapid growth. Between 2003 and 2008, nearly 3500 related papers were published in well-known clinical and research journals (Aubert & Verheyden, 2008). From this growing body of research, new findings have emerged revealing an intriguing "partnership" that apparently exists between the brain and the heart (McCraty et al., 2009). Physiological pathways used by the heart and brain when communicating have been identified, and the understanding of how these mechanisms are used by the heart to influence emotions, information processing, and perception is increasing and will, no doubt, be the focus of future research.

Practical suggestions are offered on how providers can use techniques derived from these studies to help establish, deepen, and maintain rapport with their older adult clients, patients, and customers. These simple techniques can also be used to enhance creative problem-solving, aid in decision-making, and to psychologically prepare for potentially challenging upcoming interactions, such as being in an empathic state when interacting with a frightened older adult suffering from dementia.

## THE "LITTLE BRAIN" IN THE HEART

It is well known that the human heart—approximately the size of a fist—beats about 100,000 times daily, or more than 2.5 billion times during the average life span. Six quarts of blood are circulated throughout the body about three times each minute. The body's 60,000 miles of blood vessels range in size from the aorta—the largest artery in the body (roughly the diameter of a garden hose)—to capillaries 1/10th the thickness of a human hair (Cleveland Clinic, 2014). During the average lifetime, the heart pumps the equivalent of 1,000,000 barrels of blood—enough to fill three supertankers.

What is not as well known is the knowledge that the incredible structure of the heart also includes a complex network of some 40,000 neurons, as well as various neurotransmitters and proteins similar to those found in the brain. This elaborate nervous system empowers the heart to feel, sense, encode and process information and to learn, remember, and make functional decisions independently of the cranial brain—a discovery of considerable import to providers wanting to maximize the effectiveness of the person-centered approach to communication. The heart's sophisticated nervous system qualifies it as a "little brain" (Armour, 1991; McCraty & Childre, 2002).

*The heart has its reasons which reason knows not.*

**Blaise Pascal**

## HEART–BRAIN INTERACTION AND INTERPERSONAL COMMUNICATION

Evidence suggests a complex, synergistic interaction exists between the neurons in the heart and the neurons in the brain (McCraty et al., 2009). This interaction permits the heart and brain to communicate with each other. Communication is ongoing and two-way, with each organ influencing the other. Because the heart influences brain centers involved in perception and cognitive and emotional processing, it plays an important role in the interpersonal communication process.

Evidently, the heart transmits greater amounts of information to the brain than the brain sends to the heart. For example, researchers tracking and mapping neural pathway traffic from the heart to the brain discovered much more information was flowing from the heart to the brain than was flowing from the brain to the heart (McCraty & Childre, 2010).

## HEART–BRAIN *INTRA*PERSONAL COMMUNICATION

The heart has numerous ways of communicating with the brain. Two methods—especially germane to the discussion of interpersonal communication—are the heart's rhythm and the heart's electromagnetic field (McCraty et al., 2009).

The rhythms of the heart influence the brain's ability to process information, make decisions, and solve problems, including those associated with interpersonal communication. The electromagnetic field of the heart—5000 times greater than the field generated by the brain—can be detected several feet from the body. This field extends from the body in all directions and serves as a carrier wave of information that can affect other individuals within its range. The heart signals generated by one individual can apparently affect the brain waves of another.

## HEART RATE VARIABILITY, HUMAN EMOTIONS, AND COHERENCE

Heart rate variability (HRV) measures the natural, beat-to-beat changes that occur in the heart rate (McCraty et al., 2009). The analysis of HRV is accomplished by using simple biofeedback instruments and provides an effective, noninvasive method for measuring coherence. HRV reflects the body's state of balance and stress.

When an individual experiences positive emotions such as appreciation, caring, or compassion, this is reflected in a more coherent heart rhythm. When a person experiences negative emotions such as anger or anxiety, this is reflected in an incoherent heart rhythm.

For professionals the take-away is this: When a provider genuinely experiences positive feelings such as appreciation, compassion, and love, his or her autonomic nervous system responds favorably and brain function is enhanced. This enhanced brain function results in a reduction of stress and an increase in cognitive performance conducive to the respect-based, person-centered approach to communication.

## COHERENCE AND INCOHERENCE

*Coherence* is a term that refers to the current degree of efficiency, harmony, order, and stability within a living system, such as the heart system. A coherent system is harmonious and well ordered. It reflects a balanced system running efficiently with minimal stress. An incoherent system is discordant and chaotic. It reflects an unbalanced system running inefficiently and suffering stress (Childre & Martin, 2000; McCraty et al., 2004, 2009).

The measure of coherence can indicate the degree of optimal functioning or efficiency within a system. In terms of optimal functioning, a coherent system is preferable to an incoherent system. Researchers at the Heartmath Institute™ observed that when an individual was experiencing positive emotions such as appreciation or compassion, coherence increased and a more coherent pattern of heart rhythm emerged. This pattern of coherence was identified by measuring HRV.

For providers, the important point is this: In a conversation between two or more people, an increase in one individual's heart system coherence can affect or entrain the brain waves of the others (McCraty, 2001). This entrainment process has important ramifications for establishing and maintaining rapport—the foundation of the provider–older adult relationship. Later sections of this chapter provide practical applications based on these discoveries about the heart–brain connection and offer simple techniques that can potentially enhance the quality of the provider–older adult relationship. These techniques focus on the mental activation of certain types of memories and positive emotions. This mental activation is designed to increase systemic coherence.

*Gratitude is the heart's memory.*

**French proverb**

Emotions such as genuine caring and other positive emotions (such as those associated with the person-centered approach to communication) tend to increase the patterns of coherence in heart rhythms. The resulting neural information sent to the brain facilitates cortical function.

Negative emotions such as anger, impatience, and irritability disrupt the state of coherence and create imbalance in the autonomic nervous system. These changes are reflected in disrupted heart rhythms, and the resulting neural information sent to the brain tends to impede cortical function. The net effect is that the provider of services is not providing the best care for an older adult who may be in a very vulnerable state.

## HEART-FOCUSED PRACTICAL APPLICATIONS FOR THE PROVIDER

How can a provider begin to use findings from the field of neurocardiology to enhance the interpersonal communication process? A starting point is to understand that a provider's emotions are reflected in his or her heart rhythms, and these rhythms can affect the efficiency of the provider's brain and possibly—through the process of cardioelectromagnetic communication—the brain efficiency of the older adult as well (McCraty et al., 2004, 2009). The implications of this starting point are worthy of deep contemplation and will be discussed throughout the remainder of this chapter.

As a practical application of this information, a provider with an upcoming, potentially challenging interaction with an angry, older adult suffering from Alzheimer's can increase personal coherence as a form of psychological preparation. This increase in personal coherence may result in improved cortical functioning. An increase in cortical functioning can result in increased personal awareness and a greater capacity for creative problem-solving—both in the provider and in the older adult.

Methods for increasing personal coherence are provided in this chapter. Some of the mental imagery techniques described in Chapter 8 could also be used for increasing personal systemic coherence.

To begin, providers can use the simple technique described below. It requires approximately 5–7 min to complete. Although it can be performed at any time, it may prove especially beneficial when completed immediately prior to an upcoming interaction. As an example, let us say you have an older adult as a patient who is physically slow and needs a lot of reassurance. Here is one method you can use to increase your personal heart coherence. It is similar, but not identical, to a method suggested by the Institute for Heartmath™:

1. Select a positive emotion capable of increasing personal coherence such as the feeling of deep caring, compassion, or gratitude.

2. Physically relax. Place one hand over your heart area and become aware of the sensation of your hand on your chest and especially the area of the heart beneath it.

3. Breathe naturally two to three times. Continue to breathe comfortably, but begin to imagine or pretend that you are breathing through the heart area under your hand.

4. After about a minute—using the techniques of mental imagery explained in Chapter 8—spend an additional couple of minutes vividly recollecting and re-experiencing specific memories of when you felt the selected emotion, let us say, compassion. Re-experience these feelings as vividly as possible while continuing to breathe from the heart area—aware of the heart beneath your hand. These special memories frequently involve loved ones, family, and/or friends. They often involve visits to a special place or participation in a special event or experience. These are the chocolate chip cookies of life—those special positive experiences accompanied by deeply felt positive emotions. Savor them.

5. While re-experiencing these memories and emotions, keep your general awareness in the heart area under your hand. If your mind wanders, simply bring your awareness back to the area under your hand. Continue breathing, remembering, and re-experiencing the selected emotion.

6. When finished, open your eyes. Take a few seconds to reorient yourself.

Ideally, the process of cultivating a greater state of coherence will result in enhanced cognitive functioning and decreased stress for the provider and the older adult. Hopefully, this decrease in stress combined with enhanced cognitive functioning will facilitate respectful, effective, person-centered interpersonal communication.

Several easy-to-learn techniques have been developed by the Institute for Heartmath™ for learning to purposefully evoke greater coherence. More information is available from www.Heartmath.org.

## ENERGETIC ETHICS

The provider who dwells on frustrating or unpleasant memories—who worries over what could go wrong or ruminates over what has already gone wrong, who evokes negative emotions such as anger or impatience—is a provider who is probably generating de-coherent signals from his or her heart. De-coherent heart signals can result in increased stress and decreased cognitive function—possibly for both the provider and those in close proximity. The possibility of negatively impacting those in close proximity leads once again to the principle of "do no harm"—first introduced in Chapter 2.

Although speculative, it is theoretically possible that ethical concerns may also lay within the energetic levels of interaction discussed in this chapter. Each party to a conversation emits heart signals that may influence the other, but it is the provider who carries the weight of ethical responsibility—the duty to be helpful and refrain from being harmful. As already described, evidence suggests that the heart rhythm of one person can influence the brain waves of another nearby person. A provider's emotional state has the potential to affect the state of the older adult. Theoretically, this influence can be helpful or harmful and is where the potential ethical concerns lay.

## CONCLUSION

Assuming the theories discussed in this chapter are accurate and valid, it seems the provider is in a position to exert a constructive energetic influence on the older adult or to at least refrain from doing harm. The argument offered is straightforward. When a provider chooses to dwell on positive memories, the associated positive emotions are evoked. The experience of positive emotions generates an increase in heart coherence. The state of coherence generated benefits the provider and also benefits those nearby, in this case, an older adult client. The provider's state of heart coherence can encourage increased cortical functioning in the older adult. This could prove especially beneficial when interacting with an older adult who feels anxious, angry, or afraid. The increase in heart coherence in both the provider and the older adult supports the person-centered approach to communication.

Providers can use the methods described in this chapter to better prepare for potentially challenging interactions, to evoke an increase in cortical functioning, to increase coherence, and to exert a constructive influence on those around them. In addition to the rhythms of the heart, other dimensions of subtle interpersonal interaction and influence may exist. These other dimensions will be explored in Chapter 10.

## LIST OF MAIN POINTS FOR PREVIEW AND REVIEW

- Recent research indicates interpersonal communication may be a multidimensional phenomenon.
- This chapter and the next offer speculations on how energetic-based models of human connection and interaction might influence the communication process and impact the provider–older adult relationship.
- Research suggests communication can occur between and among two or more persons via information-rich fields of electromagnetic energy.
- Studies focused on distant intentionality provide evidence that human intention can operate between individuals even when they are apart from each other.
- Neurocardiology is the specialty that deals with the brain–heart connection.
- New findings have revealed a heart–brain "partnership" that permits the heart and brain to communicate with and influence each other.
- Heart–brain interaction plays an important role in the interpersonal communication process.
- The heart includes a complex network of 40,000 neurons and various neurotransmitters and proteins similar to those found in the brain. This network empowers the heart to encode and process information, learn, remember, and make functional decisions independently of the cranial brain. The heart's sophisticated nervous system qualifies it as a "little brain."
- Heart rhythms can influence the brain's ability to process information, make decisions, and solve problems.
- The electromagnetic field of the heart can be detected several feet from the body, extends in all directions, and serves as a carrier wave of information that can affect other individuals within its range.
- Heart signals generated by one individual can affect the brain waves of another. Evidence suggests that the heart's electromagnetic field may be a source of information exchange between individuals. This exchange of information is referred to as *cardioelectromagnetic communication.*
- When two people are within conversational range, the electromagnetic signals generated by each individual's heart can influence the other person's brain rhythms.
- *Coherence* is a term that refers to the degree of efficiency, harmony, order, and stability within a living system. The measure of coherence can indicate the degree of optimal functioning or efficiency within a system.
- Coherence is measured using HRV. HRV measures beat-to-beat changes within the heart rate.

- When an individual experiences positive emotions such as appreciation, caring, or compassion, this is reflected in a coherent heart rhythm. When a person experiences negative emotions such as anger or anxiety, this is reflected as an incoherent heart rhythm.
- A provider's emotions are reflected in his or her heart rhythms. These rhythms affect the efficiency of the provider's brain and possibly the brain efficiency of the older adult as well.
- A provider can consciously increase his or her own state of heart coherence as a form of psychological preparation prior to an upcoming interaction with a patient, client, or customer. This may result in improved cortical functioning, increased personal awareness, and a greater capacity for creative problem-solving—both in the provider and in the older adult. This greater awareness encourages a more engaging and positive interaction with the older adult.
- When providers choose to dwell on positive memories and experience the associated positive emotions, they evoke beneficial effects, not only for themselves, but also for those around them.
- When providers allow themselves to dwell on negative memories and experience the associated negative emotions, they evoke undesirable effects, not only for themselves, but also for those around them.
- Providers can use techniques derived from these studies to help establish, deepen, and maintain rapport, and to help psychologically prepare for potentially challenging interactions. These techniques could prove especially beneficial when interacting with an older adult who feels anxious, angry, or afraid.

## Provider Self-Test and/or Suggestions for Instructors

**Understand key concepts:** Define and discuss *coherence, distance intentionality, electrocardiomagnetism, heart rate variability, and neurocardiology.*

**Describe:** The heart–brain partnership. Explain how these two organs interact and the impact their interaction has on each other and on the process of interpersonal communication.

**Explain:** What qualifies the heart as a "little brain."

**Discuss:** How coherence is defined and measured and the influence of coherence on the brain.

**Compare and contrast:** The effect of positive emotions versus negative emotions on the generation of coherent heart rhythms.

**Describe:** How a provider's emotions are reflected in his or her heart rhythms. Talk about how these rhythms can affect the efficiency of the provider's brain and how—during an interaction with another individual—they could influence the brain efficiency of another.

**Speculate:** Upon the potential ramifications of distance intentionality on the relationship between the provider and the older adult and on the process of establishing and maintaining professional rapport.

**Explain:** How the electromagnetic signals generated by the heart could influence the brain of another person.

**Debate and discuss:** The argument that a provider may have an ethical responsibility to evoke coherent heart rhythms prior to interaction with patients or clients.

# WEB RESOURCE

Institute of Hearthmath
www.heartmath.org

# REFERENCES

Achterberg, J., Cooke, B. S., Richards, T., Standish, L. J., Kozak, L., & Lake, J. (2005). Evidence for correlations between distant intentionality and brain function in recipients: a functional magnetic resonance imaging analysis. *Journal of Alternative and Complementary Medicine, 11*(6), 965–971.

Armour, J. A. (1991). Anatomy and function of the intrathoracic neurons regulating the mammalian heart. In I. H. Zucker, & J. P. Gilmore (Eds.), *Reflex control of the circulation* (pp. 1–37). Boca Raton, FL: CRC Press.

Aubert, A. E., & Verheyden, B. (2008). Neurocardiology: a bridge between the brain and heart. *Biofeedback, 36*(1), 15–17.

Berry, D. (2007). *Health communication: Theory and practice.* Berkshire, England: Open University Press.

Childre, D., & Martin, H. (2000). *The heartmath solution.* San Francisco, CA: Harper.

Cleveland Clinic. http://my.clevelandclinic.org/services/heart/heart-blood-vessels/heart-facts. Retrieved 14.10.14.

Combs, A., Arcari, T., & Krippner, S. (2006). All of the myriad worlds: life in the akashic plenum. *World Futures, 62,* 75–85.

Laszlo, E. (2006). *Science and the re-enchantment of the cosmos: The rise of the integral vision of reality.* Rochester, VT: Inner Traditions.

McCraty, R. (2001). *Science of the heart.* Boulder Creek. CA: Institute of Hearthmath.

McCraty, R., Atkinson, M., & Bradley, R. T. (2004). Electrophysiological evidence of intuition: part 1. The surprising role of the heart. *Journal of Alternative and Complementary Medicine, 10*(1), 133–143.

McCraty, R., Atkinson, M., Tomasino, D., & Bradley, R. T. (2009). The coherent heart, heart–brain interactions, psychophysiological coherence, and the emergence of system-wide order. *Integral Review, 5*(2), 11–114.

McCraty, R., & Childre, D. (2010). Coherence: bridging personal, social, and global health. *Alternative Therapies, 16*(4), 10–24.

McCraty, R., & Childre, D. (2002). *The appreciative heart: The psychophysiology of positive emotions and optimal functioning.* Boulder Creek, CA: Institute of HeartMath.

van der Wall, E. E. (2011). The brain–heart connection; a round trip. *Netherlands Heart Journal, 19*(6), 269–270.

CHAPTER 10

# The Physics of Interpersonal Communication: The Tenth C—Connection

*Anyone who is not shocked by quantum mechanics has not fully understood it.*
***Niels Bohr***

**Core Question:** How can a provider use information from the field of quantum physics to enhance the person-centered, interpersonal communication process?

**Keywords:** Distant intentionality; Nonlocality; Quantum entanglement.

## INTRODUCTION

Rapport, relationship, and respect are the three *R*'s of the person-centered approach to communication with older adults. Whether it is a simple smile, imagining an interaction with an older adult, or increasing the state of personal heart coherence, the methods explained in this book have one purpose—to enhance the quality of interpersonal communication. The techniques explored in this chapter are no exception. Although speculative, they offer the potential to improve the quality of interpersonal communication at the most subtle level of interaction. It may be speculated that interpersonal communication is a multidimensional process extending well beyond the simple exchange of verbal and nonverbal language. Provocative new findings continue to emerge from research into quantum mechanics, neuroscience, and consciousness studies. Several of these discoveries call for an expanded perspective of the communication process. Research findings from the field of physics offer exciting insights applicable to the understanding of interpersonal communication and human interconnection.

This chapter concludes the discussion begun in Chapter 9 and introduces the final *C—connection*. It explores theories from physics that offer fresh insights into the subtle levels of interaction that occur between individuals entangled and interconnected at the quantum level of existence (Achterberg et al., 2005;

*Person-Centered Communication with Older Adults*
http://dx.doi.org/10.1016/B978-0-12-420132-3.00010-6
**157**

Combs, Arcari, & Krippner, 2006; Laszlo, 2006; McCraty, Atkinson, Tomasino, & Bradley, 2009). The concept of quantum entanglement and interconnection may be new to many readers. Frequently, when people are first introduced to the concepts explored in this chapter, confusion is the first reaction.

Depending on the reader's background, some sections may be difficult to understand. To help increase comprehension, the key concepts will be repeated at various places. The reader is encouraged to proceed slowly, carefully ponder the concepts, and make sure they are understood before continuing. The information offered can prove helpful in expanding the provider's world view (as discussed in Chapter 2). An expanded worldview can result in improved interpersonal communication.

## THE MOST PROFOUND DISCOVERY IN ALL OF SCIENCE

Separation between individuals may be an illusion based on sensory limitations (Dossey, 2013). That may be a bold claim, but experimental evidence exists to contradict the commonly held belief that individuals are separated in space and time. After reading this chapter, each reader can decide for him or herself whether the claim is warranted.

This claim forms the philosophical foundation of this chapter and is probably the most challenging concept for providers (and nearly everyone else) to embrace. It seems counterintuitive—at odds with personal experience—esoteric pseudoscience. And, even if the claim is valid, what does it have to do with the topic of this book—person-centered communication? The remainder of this chapter is devoted to answering this question.

Despite the seeming impossibility, a plethora of empirically derived evidence is beginning to accumulate that supports this claim. Grounded in the physics concepts of *entanglement* and *nonlocality*, this conclusion may be the finding with the deepest social significance and widest range of implications regarding human interconnection. Henry Stapp—a theoretical physicist at the University of California-Berkeley—characterized nonlocality as the "most profound discovery in all of science" (Dossey, 2011a, p. 337).

Elaborating on the significance of this discovery, Dossey, (2011a) exclaimed, "This realization will profoundly affect our concept of our place in the universe and what it means to be human" (p. 336). Larry Dossey, MD, is the author of 12 books and numerous articles. Dossey is the former executive editor of the peer-reviewed journal *Alternative Therapies in Health and Medicine* and is currently executive editor of the peer-reviewed journal *Explore: The Journal of Science and Healing.*

Deep human interconnection is not a new concept. Dean Radin, Ph.D. (2006) explains, "For thousands of years it's been one of the core assumptions underlying Eastern philosophies. What is new, is that Western science is slowly beginning to realize that some elements of an ancient lore might have been correct" (p. 3).

This chapter discusses three pathways that may be involved with the process of interconnection—*nonlocality, quantum entanglement,* and *distance intentionality*—concepts borrowed from the field of physics. Providers are encouraged to consider how integration of these concepts into their professional worldview could impact the person-centered approach to service delivery.

## DISTANCE BENEVOLENT INTENTION

Many individuals—providers or not—regularly engage in small acts of benevolent mental intention. What is a benevolent mental intention? Prayers and blessing are two obvious examples. Additional examples include mentally sending "get well" wishes to an ailing family member or friend, wishing someone good luck, or keeping fingers crossed for a friend being interviewed for a new job (Schmidt, 2012). All of these examples could be characterized as expressions of benevolent mental intention—distance intentionality.

In the past, most researchers routinely dismissed scientific inquiries into distance intentionality—benevolent or otherwise. The concept of human intention influencing someone or something from a distance did not seem to fit with the then current scientific paradigm. Eventually, the sheer amount of evidence that supported distant mental influence or intentionality made it impossible to ignore any longer, and the scientific community began showing an increased interest in its study (Achterberg et al., 2005). As Dossey (2013) reminds, the deliberate exclusion of crucial scientific evidence is a form of scientific malpractice (p. 6).

## DISTANCE INTENTIONALITY

Distance intention refers to the concept that human intention can impact the physical world and other humans from a distance. Studies focused on the phenomenon of distant intentionality provide overwhelming evidence that human intention can impact and influence individuals (and other forms of matter) from a distance (Achterberg et al., 2005).

The lead researcher of the previously referenced article was the late Jeanne Achterberg—an internationally recognized scientist acclaimed for her pioneering work in medicine and psychology. Author of more than 100 papers and five books, she also co-chaired the mind/body interventions ad hoc advisory panel and the Research Technologies Conference of the Office of Alternative Medicine and served as senior editor for the peer-reviewed *Journal of Alternative Therapies.*

Hundreds of studies have been conducted that support the concept of distant intention (Zahourek, 2004). Dossey (1982) described a meta-analysis of 832 studies that indicated people could influence random processes. He stated the odds against chance accounting for the significant results of this meta-analysis were greater than one trillion to one.

Nonlocal, distant communication has been repeatedly demonstrated from multiple areas of research. These areas include findings from studies exploring distance healing—influence from person-to-person, brain-to-brain, and neurons-to-neurons (Dossey, 2013; Schlitz & Radin, 2008). In each example, the objects (although physically separated) behaved as if they were a single entity—as if they were nonlocally connected. From the perspective of traditional science, none of these interactions should be possible. It bears repeating that these experimental effects are often small, yet statistically significant.

Credible evidence from multiple sources supports the conclusion that it is possible for one individual (the influencer) to influence the thoughts, feelings, behaviors, and physiological and physical activities of other individuals and other organisms (the influenced)—even when the two are separated and beyond the reach of conventional senses (Braud, 2003).

## THE CENTRAL INTELLIGENCE AGENCY AND DISTANCE INTENTION

From the early 1970s through the early 1990s, the United States Central Intelligence Agency was involved in research exploring the potential of nonlocal consciousness and distance intention. They established the Stanford Research Institute (SRI) in California—led by physicist Russell Targ—to investigate this potential. Thousands of experiments were conducted. Commonly referred to as remote viewing, these studies—using distance mental intention—explored whether this phenomena could be used for gathering intelligence from a distance, in other words, spying (Wayne, 2006).

For those desiring additional information, several books were published after this project was declassified and disbanded. Although speculative, the evidence gathered at the Stanford Research Institute lends additional support to the argument that a provider and older adult may be able to exert a least a small amount of mutual influence. If providers exert any distance influence whatsoever, they are encouraged to exert benevolent influence.

## Experiment

Objective: Combine the exercise for increasing heart coherence (explained in Chapter 9) with knowledge of the concepts of energetic human interconnection and distance intentionality from this chapter to help psychologically prepare for a challenging upcoming interaction with an older adult.

1. Select a positive emotion demonstrated to increase personal coherence such as the feeling of deep caring, compassion, or gratitude.
2. Physically relax for a couple of minutes.
3. Place one hand over your heart area and become aware of the feeling of your hand on your chest and especially the area of the heart beneath it. Breathe naturally two to three times.
4. Continue to breathe comfortably, but begin to imagine or pretend that you are breathing through the heart area underneath your hand.
5. After about a minute—using the techniques of mental imagery explained in Chapter 8—spend a short time vividly recollecting and re-experiencing specific memories of when you had a positive interaction with an older adult and feel the emotion. Re-experience these feelings as vividly as possible while continuing to breathe from the heart area—aware of the heart beneath your hand. These special memories frequently involve loved ones, family, and/or friends. While re-experiencing these memories and emotions, keep your general awareness in the heart area under your hand. If your mind wanders, simply bring your awareness back to the area under your hand.
6. Continue breathing, remembering, and re-experiencing the selected emotion. Using your imagination, picture the person with whom you are planning to meet.
7. Spend a couple of minutes contemplating the concepts of human interconnection and distance intentionality—especially the connection between you and the potentially challenging older adult. Imagine that you may be able to help this older adult feel more comfortable by increasing your own personal comfort.
8. Using your imagination, mentally discuss your concerns with the person you plan to meet. Visualize the interaction proceeding constructively and ending positively. When finished, open your eyes. Take a few seconds to reorient yourself.

## ADVANCES IN RESEARCH INTO DISTANCE INTENTIONALITY

Research into distance intentionality has progressed significantly. Carefully planned, tightly controlled, highly sophisticated studies of distance intentionality have now been conducted utilizing functional magnetic resonance imaging technology for gathering data. These studies—along with many others—generated empirical evidence of correlative activity between the brain functions of two individuals that were physically separated. When the brain of one person was stimulated in a certain way, evidence of that stimulation appeared instantly in the brain of the other person (Achterberg et al., 2005).

Because no known processes can account for this correlative brain activity, the results can be interpreted as producing evidence of entanglement and distant intentionality (Achterberg et al., 2005). Studies such as these support the conclusion that human intentions may directly affect other individuals by unknown mechanisms. This finding highlights the theoretical possibility that a provider's thoughts, images, and emotions might be able to function as a nontraditional mode for expressing caring concern, compassion, empathy, and encouragement—as a means for providing nonlocal, person-centered encouragement.

### Summary

Quantum entanglement refers to the concept that two objects, once in contact, remain in contact. This contact is unaffected by distance. When objects are entangled, a change in one object produces an immediate change in the other object—a change that requires no time, no known means of connection, and that occurs instantly no matter how great the physical separation. This instant communication is referred to as nonlocality. Quantum entanglement is the state or condition. Nonlocality is the process. In other words, nonlocal communication between distant entities is instantaneous, unmediated by any known energetic signal, and unmitigated in that it does not appear to diminish with increasing distance (Herbert, 1987). What does it mean that a provider and older adult are energetically interconnected? How can understanding this interconnection enhance the communication process? Providers are encouraged to contemplate these questions as they explore the remainder of this chapter.

## DEVELOPMENT OF QUANTUM MECHANICS AND ENTANGLEMENT

Until the early 1900s—during the pre-quantum era of physics—it was commonly assumed that the world "out there" existed in a well-defined, relatively fixed state, irrespective of whether, how, or by whom it was observed. As the twentieth century unfolded, experimental findings from contemporary physicists began to suggest (and later demonstrate) this view to be inaccurate. In its stead, they offered the intriguing possibility of a world in which the observer and the observed are inextricably interwoven and mutually influencing (Davies & Gribbon, 1992; Walach, 2005).

When the previous sentence above is modified so the terms *observer* and *observed* are replaced with the terms *provider* and *older adult*, provocative, yet practical speculations are possible. Here is the modified sentence: Experimental findings from contemporary quantum physicists suggest the intriguing possibility of a world in which the provider and the older adult are inextricably interwoven and mutually influencing. This concept of mutually influential interweaving—a type of *entanglement*—has the potential to transform the common understanding of cause and effect and perspectives on interconnection, relationships, and interpersonal communication.

Quantum mechanics developed in the early twentieth century, mostly through the efforts of such notables as Albert Einstein, Niels Bohr, Werner Heisenberg, Erwin Schrodinger, and others (Radin, Storm, & Tressoldi, 2010). Quantum mechanics is traditionally described as a theory of microscopic things. Recently, more and more physicists have taken the position that quantum mechanics applies to all things—microscopic and macroscopic—even human beings (Vedral, 2011). This shift in scientific attitude is important. It means many researchers are admitting the possibility that the concept of entanglement may apply to people.

## ENTANGLEMENT

The concept of *entanglement*—borrowed from quantum theory—predicts that "under certain circumstances particles that appear to be isolated are actually instantaneously connected through time and space" (Radin, 2005, p. 11). This means that even though atomic particles are physically separated, they behave as if they are connected—a change in one results in an instantaneous change in the other—a phenomena that has been repeatedly confirmed. Radin is Chief Scientist for the Institute of Noetic Sciences. Author of over 200 articles, a dozen book chapters, and three books, he has been engaged in research on the nature of consciousness for more than 20 years (http://www.deanradin.com/NewWeb/bio.html).

Evidence continues to mount pointing to the conclusion that objects (and perhaps people) are energetically interconnected (entangled) at the subatomic, quantum level of existence (Achterberg et al., 2005; Combs et al., 2006; Laszlo, 2006; McCraty et al., 2009). This conclusion troubled

Albert Einstein. In a 1947 letter to physicist Max Born, Einstein characterized quantum mechanics and entanglement as "spooky action at a distance." Despite Einstein's historical objections, quantum mechanics and its actions at a distance now enjoy wide acceptance and are commonly referred to as nonlocality (Leder, 2005).

Although the subatomic connections between objects are unseen, the research is sometimes speculative, and some of the implications are controversial; these findings make the possibility very real that providers can subtly communicate with and influence older adults—even from a distance. As bizarre as this may sound to some, there is significant evidence to support the concept of nonlocal (at a distance) influence (Greene, 2007). Exactly, *how* this nonlocal interconnection takes place, remains unknown. The reader is once again encouraged to contemplate the implications of this concept in terms of interpersonal communication and person-centered service delivery.

## ENTANGLED HUMAN BEINGS

According to quantum theory—and repeated, replicated experimental studies—the connection between atomic particles can persist no matter how far they are physically separated. This means exactly what it implies. It means that if two particles that had once been in contact and are now entangled are each sent in opposite directions, that no matter how far apart they may be, at an energetic level, they remain in constant, immediate contact. A change in one particle results in the *instantaneous* change in the other. Readers struggling with accepting the possibility of this phenomena are in good company—many physicists who fully embrace the reality of this concept, still struggle with its implications.

Although robust evidence exists to support the conclusion that nonlocal interconnections (quantum entanglements) exist at the subatomic level of existence, connection at the level of human-to-human (generalized quantum entanglement) is still being debated (Hyland, 2003). Tiller, Dibble, and Fandel (2005) provided summaries of experimental support that demonstrated the possibility of energy/information entanglement between objects, between humans, and between humans and objects. Lanza and Berman (2009) speculated, "it may even make sense that everything is in some sense an entangled relative of every other, and in direct contact with everything else, despite the seeming emptiness between them" (p. 125).

Arguments continue over the theoretical difficulties of maintaining quantum entanglement at the human level. But, as Schlitz and Radin remarked in Millay's (2010) book, *Radiant Minds*, "one cannot help wondering, what if this concept *did* apply to humans" (p. 105).

## Summary—Revisited

To aid reader comprehension and learning, the summary presented earlier in this chapter is repeated again here. Quantum entanglement refers to the concept that two objects, once in contact, remain in contact. This contact is unaffected by distance. When objects are entangled, a change in one object produces an immediate change in the other object—a change that requires no time, no known means of connection, and that occurs instantly no matter how great the physical separation. This instant communication is referred to as nonlocality. Quantum entanglement is the state or condition. Nonlocality is the process. In other words, nonlocal communication between distant entities is instantaneous, unmediated by any known energetic signal, and unmitigated in that is does not appear to diminish with increasing distance (Herbert, 1987).

Entanglement demonstrates the physical world—at the microscopic level and quite possibly at all levels—works in ways very different from the commonly accepted views about cause and effect. At this point, this chapter's opening quote also bears repeating,

*Anyone who is not shocked by quantum mechanics has not fully understood it.*
*Niels Bohr*

# THE INTERACTION OF CONSCIOUSNESS AND MATTER

Some of the breakthrough findings that demonstrated how human consciousness could interact with and influence the physical world first derived from experimentation with electrons. Physicists postulate that the physical world is constructed out of elementary particles called electrons (Davies & Gribbon, 1992; Walach, 2005).

Evidently, these electrons—the subatomic building blocks of all physical existence—can behave as both waves and particles depending how they are observed or measured. How do physicists explain this?

Apparently, electrons that are unobserved behave differently than electrons that are being watched or measured. When electrons are not being observed or measured, they behave as probability fields—waves having no precise location. But when electrons are being observed or measured, the probability fields collapse into fixed particles that can now be located in a particular place. Whether electrons exist as fields of probability or actual particles seems to depend on the presence of an observing consciousness (Davies & Gribbon, 1992). The implication is clear:

> *It Appears that Human Consciousness Can Interact with and Influence the Fabric of Existence.*

Readers are encouraged to contemplate this last sentence. The ability of consciousness to influence physical matter has been repeatedly demonstrated in experiments using diverse subjects. Braud (1994) explained, "Statistically significant remote mental influences have been observed in experiments with bacteria, fungus colonies, yeast, plants, protozoa, larvae, wood lice, aunts, fish, chicks, mice, rats, gerbils, cats, dogs, dolphins, and humans" (p. 67). This influencing observer effect is not based on some hocus-pocus. The effects may be small, but they are real.

This chapter has explored how these esoteric-sounding, yet laboratory-based research findings might influence the practical, day-to-day interactions of a provider and the older adults he or she serves. Using various examples and explanations that approach the topic from different perspectives, the same point has been repeatedly made—empirical evidence suggests that person-to-person, mutually influential interconnection is highly probable.

## BELL'S THEOREM ON NONLOCALITY

Bell's theorem is viewed as one of the most profound breakthrough developments of physics (Brunner, Cavalcanti, Pironio, Scarani, & Wehner, 2014). Bell's theorem on nonlocality—which has been empirically validated and repeatedly replicated—introduced the concept that everything in the known universe behaves as if it is connected to everything else and that nonlocal interaction between particles is instantaneous and not affected by distance (Davies & Gribbon, 1992; Dossey, 1982). Essentially, Bell's theorem postulates that there is no such thing as actual physical separation.

Speculative interpretations of Bell's theorem—combined with evidence from studies of quantum entanglement—lend theoretical support to the concept that once a provider and an older adult interact, some of the atoms of each person will have become permanently intertwined (entangled) at the quantum level of existence (Radin, 2006; Walach, 2005). Bell's theorem also offers the intriguing possibility that the comingled atoms of the provider and older adult will continue to affect one another although seemingly physically separated. Lanza and Berman (2009) concluded that, "Bell's experiment implies that there are cause–effect linkages that transcend our ordinary classical way of thinking" (p. 183).

## HUMAN–MACHINE INTERACTION ANOMALIES

Dossey (2011b) described research conducted by Radin and Nelson. Evidently, these researchers analyzed over 800 studies that examined the effect of human intention on random number generators. Their findings provided reliable, replicable evidence for direct mental influence on randomly generated events.

Even more impressive, experiments conducted by the Princeton Engineering Laboratory focused on the anomalies of human–machine interaction. Over a 28-year period of time, thousands of experiments were conducted involving millions of trials and hundreds of participants. The objective of the participants was to use mental intention to attempt to influence various acoustical, electronic, mechanical, and optical devices that normally produce an output of purely random data.

The studies generated a massive quantity of empirical evidence demonstrating small (but statistically significant) changes in the output of these devices—changes that can only be attributed to the mental influence of the participants (http://www.princeton.edu/~pear/experiments.html). These experiments strongly suggest that "consciousness has the ability to bias probabilistic systems" (Jahn & Dunne, 2009, p. xii).

This section—similar to many others in this chapter—offered empirically grounded examples to support the argument that providers and older adults (and all other people) live in a world of deep, underlying interconnection—a world where conscious intention can exert a small but real influence on one another. It is possible that this minute influence could be used to help or harm. For example, it is common for providers to have thoughts and feelings about their older adult clients, residents, or patients—especially just before or immediately following an interaction. Providers sometimes talk with colleagues about their clients. These conversations might occur with a supervisor, other involved providers, or at a staff meeting.

The main argument of this chapter is that enough research has been accumulated to suggest that—no matter how small the effect—the thoughts and words shared about an older adult may have a greater influence than was previously believed. If this is true, then—for the sake of the older adults served—it would behoove providers to remain mindful of the potential impact of their thoughts and words. The next section offers an example illustrating what might be, based on a real incident.

Mary, a nurse working at an assisted living facility, was tired. She had already been on the job—and on her feet—for 8 h when the call buzzer from the resident in room #36 began to sound. Room #36 was Betty's room. Yes, Betty had a tendency to push the help button a little too often. She was nearing 90, felt afraid much of the time, and was in need of frequent emotional reassurance.

Mary, the nurse on this shift, was behind in her charting, plus she had two other residents who also needed her attention. Feeling tired and frustrated, with a heavy sigh, Mary blurted out to no one in particular, "What the hell does that old bag of skin and bones want now? She is always talking about dying. God, I wish she'd just die and get on with it!"

Imagine that Mary and Betty live in a world of deep interconnection, a world where information is instantly exchanged via deep pathways of energetic connection. Imagine Betty lives in a world where at some level of her being—a level outside her conscious awareness—she is receiving the message from Mary, "God, I wish she'd just die and get on with it!" If you were Betty, how would you feel?

Nurse Mary may have responded differently to Betty's call had she been aware of several clinical studies that confirmed distance benevolent human intention could be correlated with specific desirable outcomes in target participants (Schmidt, 2012). If Mary had known of those studies, she might have realized the opposite may also hold true—harmful intentions may be correlated with specific undesirable outcomes. The implication is clear: Evidence suggests that it is possible for providers to exert a constructive influence on older adults by thinking, speaking, and behaving toward them in a constructive and life-affirming manner—whether in their physical presence or separated.

## ETHICAL CONCERNS REVISITED

The principle of "do no harm" was first introduced in Chapter 2. It was revisited in Chapter 9 and now again in this chapter. The argument offered throughout these chapters is straightforward. Via a number of evidence-based pathways or mechanisms (heart rhythms, electromagnetic fields, quantum entanglement, nonlocality, and distance intentionality), it is possible that ethical concerns may extend into the subtle, less tangible domains of interaction.

The theories, concepts, and evidence presented in this chapter suggest the provider is in a position to exert a small, but real energetic influence on the older adult. If this is accurate, then it is the provider's duty and responsibility to at least attempt to exert a helpful influence and refrain from exerting a harmful influence.

Evidence indicates that human interaction and interconnection occur that are clearly beyond conventionally accepted limits. An individual's mental influence is able to interact with another person from a distance. The potential social implications are profound. Previously confined to the domains of philosophy, metaphysics, and mysticism, the concept that the universe is interconnected is now being taken seriously by increasing numbers of scientists and researchers.

So much evidence for a deep, underlying interconnection between people exists, that as Braud (1994) described, "It is difficult to understand how such anomalous interaction could occur if an underlying matrix of subtle yet important connections among people did not exist" (p. 70).

In the face of substantial evidence pointing to human entanglement, Larry Dossey, MD encourages everyone to courageously embrace this realization of essential oneness and allow it to shape how we live our lives. With respect to the person-centered approach to interpersonal communication, he wisely suggests, "What we commonly call empathy, compassion, and love may be human entanglement banging on the doors of consciousness to gain entry" (Dossey, 2011, p. 343).

## CONCLUSION

One objective of this chapter was to invite providers to consider the possibility that human energetic interconnection may indeed be a fact; to integrate awareness of this very real possibility into their professional world view; and finally, to think, speak, and behave accordingly. For example, holding this view of subtle universal interconnection may prove helpful when interacting with an angry older adult suffering from age-related hearing loss and dementia. It may help the provider to be better able to access his or her feelings of compassion and empathy and from that perspective, communicate in a manner that reflects the seven C's—caring, compassionate, courteous, clear, concise, congruent, and complete.

Here is an example that illustrates how to turn theory into practice. A provider (who has completed study of this chapter) is one day preparing for an upcoming interaction with a difficult client. The provider pauses to think, "I don't really know if all that stuff about nonlocal connection and distance intentionality is true or not. But, there seems to be enough evidence to at least suggest it's possible. So, just in case, I'm going to 'send' this client some mental encouragement—let him know that I respect and care about him."

## LIST OF MAIN POINTS FOR PREVIEW AND REVIEW

- This chapter extends and concludes the exploration begun in Chapter 9 of the more subtle dynamics and pathways of interpersonal communication.
- Three new potential pathways from physics are discussed: nonlocality, distance intentionality, and quantum entanglement.
- Experimental evidence strongly suggests human isolation is an illusion.
- Evidence points to the conclusion that people are energetically interconnected (entangled) at the subatomic, quantum level of existence.
- The concept of *entanglement* predicts that under certain circumstances particles that appear to be isolated are actually instantaneously connected through time and space.
- These findings make very real the possibility that providers can subtly communicate with and influence older adults—even from a distance.
- Studies focused on the phenomenon of distant intentionality provide overwhelming evidence that human intention can impact and influence individuals (and other forms of matter) from a distance.
- Experimental findings from quantum physicists suggest the possibility of a world in which the provider and the older adult are inextricably interwoven and mutually influencing.
- Although robust evidence exists to support the conclusion that nonlocal interconnections exist at the subatomic level of existence, connection at the level of human-to-human (generalized quantum entanglement) remains under debate.
- Entanglement demonstrates the physical world—at least at the subatomic level—works in ways very different from the commonly accepted views about cause and effect.
- Bell's theorem on nonlocality introduced the concept that everything in the known universe behaves as if it is connected to everything else and

that nonlocal interaction between particles is instantaneous and not affected by distance. Essentially, Bell's theorem postulates that there is no such thing as actual physical separation.

- Distance intention refers to the concept that human intention can impact matter from a distance. Nonlocal, distant communication has been repeatedly demonstrated from multiple areas of research. Hundreds of studies have been conducted that support the concept of distant intention.
- Experiments strongly suggest that consciousness has the ability to bias probabilistic systems.
- This chapter offered empirically derived evidence that can be interpreted to support the argument that providers and older adults (and all other people) live in a world of deep, underlying interconnection—a world where conscious intention can exert a small but real influence on another.
- Research is beginning to accumulate suggesting that thoughts and words shared about an older adult may have a greater influence than is commonly believed.
- Dozens of studies support the conclusion that human intentions may directly affect others via unknown mechanisms.
- One objective of this chapter is to invite providers to consider that human energetic interconnection may indeed be a fact; to integrate awareness of this very real possibility into their professional world view; and finally, to think, speak, and behave accordingly.
- The evidence could be interpreted to support the argument that a provider and older adult may be able to exert mutual influence from a distance.
- The argument offered throughout these chapters is straightforward. Via a number of evidence-based pathways or mechanisms—heart rhythms, electromagnetic fields, quantum entanglement, nonlocality and distance intentionality—it is possible that ethical concerns may extend into the subtle, less tangible domains of interaction.
- The theories, concepts, and evidence presented in this chapter suggest that the provider is in a position to exert a small, but real energetic influence on the older adult. If this is accurate, then it is the provider's duty and responsibility to attempt to exert a helpful influence and refrain from exerting a harmful influence.
- Providers are encouraged to courageously embrace a realization of essential oneness and allow this realization to shape their thoughts, words, and actions.

## Provider Self-Test and/or Suggestions for Instructors

**Understand key concepts:** Define and discuss *distance intentionality, nonlocality,* and *quantum entanglement.*

**Discuss:** What it means that a provider and older adult are energetically interconnected.

**Discuss:** How can understanding this interconnection enhance the communication process?

**Debate:** The pros and cons of the argument that a provider's ethical responsibility to do no harm extends into the nontangible, subtle domains of energetic interconnection.

# WEB RESOURCES

## Journals

Explore: The Journal of Science and Healing
   http://www.explorejournal.com/issues
Journal of Nonlocality
   http://journals.sfu.ca/jnonlocality/index.php/jnonlocality/index

## People

Jeanne Achterberg
   http://www.jeanneachterberg.com/index.html
Larry Dossey
   http://larrydosseymd.com/
Dean Dean Radin
   http://www.deanradin.com/NewWeb/deanradin.html

## Organizations

Institute of Noetic Sciences
   http://noetic.org/
The Princeton Engineering Anomalies Research (PEAR)
   http://www.princeton.edu/~pear/

# REFERENCES

Achterberg, J., Cooke, K., Richards, T., Standish, L. J., Kozak, L., & Lake, J. (2005). Evidence for correlations between distant intentionality and brain function in recipients: a functional magnetic resonance imaging analysis. *The Journal of Alternative and Complementary Medicine, 11*(6), 965–971.

Braud, W. (1994). Empirical exploration of prayer, distance healing, and remote influence. *The Journal of Religion and Psychical Research, 17*(2), 62–73.

Braud, W. (2003). *Distant mental influence: Its contributions to science, healing, and human interactions.* Charlottesville, VA: Hampton Roads Publishing.

Brunner, N., Cavalcanti, D., Pironio, S., Scarani, V., & Wehner, S. (2014). Bell's nonlocality. *Reviews of Modern Physics, 86*(2), 419–478.

Combs, A., Arcari, T., & Krippner, S. (2006). All of the myriad worlds: life in the akashic plenum. *World Futures, 62*, 75–85.

Davies, P., & Gribbon, J. (1992). *The matter myth: Dramatic discoveries that challenge our understanding of physical reality*. New York: Simon and Schuster.

Dossey, L. (1982). *Space, time & medicine*. London: Shambhala.

Dossey, L. (2011a). All tangled up: life in a quantum world. *Explore, 7*(6), 335–344.

Dossey, L. (2011b). *Healing words*. Kindle. Harper Collins.

Dossey, L. (2013). Unbroken wholeness: the emerging view of human interconnection. *Explore, 9*(1), 1–8.

Greene, B. (2007). *The fabric of the cosmos: Space, time, and the texture of reality*. New York: Random House.

Herbert, N. (1987). *Quantum reality*. Garden City, NY: Doubleday.

Hyland, M. E. (2003). Extended network generalized entanglement theory: therapeutic mechanisms, empirical predictions, and investigations. *The Journal of Alternative and Complementary Medicine, 9*(6), 919–936.

Jahn, R. G., & Dunne, B. J. (2009). *Margins of reality: The role of consciousness in the physical world*. Princeton, NJ: ICRL Press.

Lanza, R., & Berman, B. (2009). *Biocentrism: How life and consciousness are the keys to understanding the true nature of the universe*. Dallas, TX: BanBella.

Laszlo, E. (2006). *Science and the re-enchantment of the cosmos: The rise of the integral vision of reality*. Rochester, VT: Inner Traditions.

Leder, D. (2005). "Spooky actions at a distance": physics, psi, and distant healing. *Journal of Alternative & Complementary Medicine, 11*(5), 923–930.

McCraty, R., Atkinson, M., Tomasino, D., & Bradley, R. T. (2009). The coherent heart, heart-brain interactions, psychophysiological coherence, and the emergence of system-wide order. *Integral Review, 5*(2), 1–115.

Millay, J. (Ed.). (2010). *Radiant minds: Scientists explore the dimensions of consciousness*. Doyle, CA: Millay. Princeton Engineering Anomalies Research. http://www.princeton.edu/~pear/.

Radin, D. (2005). *Entangled minds. Shift: At the frontiers of consciousness, December 2004–February 2005*. 11–14.

Radin, D. (2006). *Entangled minds*. New York: Simon and Schuster.

Radin, D., Storm, L., & Tressoldi, P. E. (2010). Extrasensory perception and quantum models of cognition. *NeuroQuantology, 8*(4), 81–87.

Schlitz, M., & Radin, D. (2008). *Prayer and intention in distant healing in measuring the measurable*. Boulder, CO: Soundstrue.

Schmidt, S. (2012). Can we help just by good intentions? A meta-analysis of experiments on distant intention effects. *The Journal of Alternative and Complementary Medicine, 18*(6), 529–533.

Tiller, W. A., Dibble, W. E., & Fandel, J. G. (2005). *Some science adventures with real magic*. Walnut Creek, CA: Pavior.

Vedral, V. (2011). Living in a quantum world. *Scientific American, 304*, 38–43.

Walach, H. (2005). Generalized entanglement: a new theoretical model for understanding the effects of complementary and alternative medicine. *The Journal of Alternative and Complementary Medicine, 11*(3), 549–559.

Wayne, M. (2006). Consciousness and nonlocality. *Alternative Therapies, 12*(6), 64–67.

Zahourek, Rothlyn (November/December 2004). Intentionality forms the matrix of healing: a theory. *Alternative Therapies, 10*, 40–49.

CHAPTER 11

# Person-Centered Interpersonal Communications: The Future of Aging

*Prediction is very difficult, especially if it's about the future.*

*Niels Bohr*

**Core Question:** How might a person-centered, interpersonal communication approach benefit the providers and older adults of the high-tech future?

**Keywords:** Forecast; Fusion; Internet of Things; Nanotechnology; Prediction; Trends.

## INTRODUCTION

This chapter attempts to provide a glimpse of elders of the past, present, and future. Although the society of the future will probably look and feel very different than today's society, providers trained in person-centered interpersonal communication will almost certainly continue to play a significant role.

This chapter offers "educated guesses" about what the future may hold for the projected 1.5 billion elders of 2050. It emphasizes the benefits a person-centered communication approach could bring to the 59 million providers who will assist them. Whether 2014 or 2030, effective, person-centered communication will most likely remain essential to the successful provider–older adult professional relationship.

## HUMANITY'S FAMILY TREE: THE ELDERS OF PAST, PRESENT, AND FUTURE

From the time of the first human up through the year 2014, approximately 100 billion people have lived on earth. These are the past and present members of humanity's family tree. The current population of over seven billion have genetic roots extending back through approximately 93 billion ancestors.

By 2050, the earth's population is expected to exceed nine billion. At that time, one out of every five persons will be aged 65 or older and—for

*Person-Centered Communication with Older Adults*
http://dx.doi.org/10.1016/B978-0-12-420132-3.00011-8

the first time in history—the number of older adults will exceed those aged 15 or younger (World Health Organization, 2011).

In 2009, a medical journal—*The Lancet*—projected that most babies born since 2000 in countries identified as having populations with long life expectancies (the United States, Canada, Japan, France, Germany, Italy, and the United Kingdom) will live to celebrate their 100th birthday (Christensen, Doblhammer, Rau, & Vaupel, 2009). They will be the elders of the future.

## THE CHANGING ROLE OF THE ELDER

Currently, there are approximately 531 million elders (individuals aged 65 or older)—a number predicted to double by 2030 and reach over 1.5 billion by 2050 (World Health Organization, 2011). Throughout much of history—up until the Industrial Revolution which took place from the eighteenth to nineteenth centuries—elders were routinely held in high esteem. Often occupying the more honored roles of society such as judges and social leaders, elders were considered to be the sages and seers—the gatekeepers of social order and the guardians of tradition.

Instructors of the next generation, the elders were frequently viewed as the wise ones (Schachter-Shalomi & Miller, 1995). With the dawn of the Industrial Revolution and its increasing emphasis on technological knowledge, "elders lost their esteemed place in society and fell into the disempowered state that we now ascribe to a 'normal' old age" (Schachter-Shalomi & Miller, 1995, p. 6).

## THE FUTURE: SOME THINGS CHANGE, SOME DO NOT

Few claims about the future can be made with certainty. What is fairly certain is that in the decades to come (barring catastrophic global disasters), there will be more elders than at any other time in history, and this generation of older adults will differ in significant ways from previous generations, for example, more years of education and smaller family size (Robnett & Chop, 2010). Unlike the preceding generation, the new elders typically view themselves as partners with their providers, routinely assume an active role in service planning, make their own informed decisions, and they insist on being treated with courtesy, compassion, and respect.

Communication occurs within a relationship. Relationships have a timeless value—always in style. Relationships emerge over time as a result of interpersonal communication. Without some type of communication, there is no relationship.

In the future, the older adult may be at home standing in front of a wall-sized screen consulting with the digital image of a virtual medical doctor or physically present for a dental appointment and sitting in the dentist's chair. In either scenario, the elder of the future will almost certainly prefer working with an empathic provider who treats him or her with respect—a professional committed to a person-centered approach to communication guided by the 10 C's—caring, compassionate, courteous, clear, concise, congruent, complete, calm, coherent, and connected. These timeless characteristics of high-quality communication are not likely to go out of fashion.

Some things do not change much. A core argument of this book has been that—within the context of a widely diverse aging services network—effective communication is essential to the successful provider–older adult professional relationship. It is reasonable to assert that this claim *was* historically valid, *is* presently valid, and in the foreseeable future, it *will* continue to be valid.

Respect-based, person-centered communication is not an old-fashioned concept. Whether the year is 2014 or 2030, improved communication can help form meaningful professional relationships, deepen rapport, increase mutual respect and understanding, and enhance the accurate exchange of information. It can improve compliance with provider recommendations, positively impact service outcomes, and often save time—all this while lowering frustration and stress for both the provider and the older adult.

The older adult of the future will likely be educated, empowered, engaged, equipped, and enabled, and he or she will expect the provider to treat him or her accordingly (Mesko, 2014a). Effective, respectful communication skills will be in high demand.

## THE FIVE BARRIERS TO EFFECTIVE COMMUNICATION—REVISITED

The five barriers to effective, mutually satisfying communication (described in Chapter 1) will most likely continue to play a role in future provider–older adult interactions. Although improvement in these areas is progressing, much more is anticipated. These five barriers (plus additional comments) include the following:

1. *Underdeveloped professional communication skills.* More and more attention is being paid to this barrier. There is growing recognition that effective communication is a core, professional skill set. Within various provider circles, gradual and steady improvement is occurring that should continue into the future. Increasing numbers of high-quality communication

training programs are available across a wide range of learning platforms. These platforms include audio CDs, DVDs, Web sites, streaming video series, webinars, webcasts, podcasts, smartphone and computer apps, university-sponsored continuing education programs, weekend workshops, certificate programs, and other hybrid trainings offered by related professional organizations. Changes have been made to the curriculum of certain provider training programs requiring completion of a course in communication. Both the Accreditation Council on Graduate Medical Education and the American Board of Medical Specialties have identified communication skill as a core competency (National Institute on Aging, 2011). The Joint Commission, which accredits hospitals, instructed hospitals to "make effective communication a priority for patient safety" (Robnett & Chop, 2010). These are some of the changes already in effect that should encourage ongoing development of provider communication skills.

2. *Lack of commitment to a person-centered service delivery system.* Members of the baby boom generation will likely demand more personalized professional services than did the previous generation. Some of the regulatory bodies and payor sources associated with the aging services network are issuing new directives aimed at providers that encourage (or require) integration of evidence-based methods and techniques into their service delivery process—including person-centered service. The United States Institute of Medicine listed respectful, person-centered care as one of the necessary features required for delivery of high-quality care. These combined pressures could help accelerate the widespread adoption of the person-centered approach. There are many high-tech advancements soon expected. These include personalized medicine, in-home virtual medical visits, robotic personal care assistants, and the use of advanced remote sensors to help monitor factors associated with aging in place. These technological advancements will require a "high-touch" communication approach to help older adults better understand the purpose, process, and day-to-day operation and maintenance of these new systems and tools. When the technical side of service becomes even more complex, the need for the person-centered, clinical side of service will become even more important.

3. *Inappropriate use of professional jargon.* Several influential forces are converging that should result in the continued reduction in the use of overly complex, technical, professional jargon. The ongoing demand placed on providers by the baby boomers for clear, concise communication, combined with the changes associated with barrier number 1, and the

increasing adoption of plain language standards by various regulatory, payor, and publishing sources should help decrease unnecessary use of confusing, overly technical jargon.

4. *Ageist attitudes and language.* Influence exerted on providers by members of the baby boom generation; changes in the way mass media depicts older adults; zero-tolerance policies of various licensing and regulatory bodies; combined with an increase in mandatory diversity training for providers and the changes associated with barrier number 1 should help to reduce ageist attitudes and use of ageist language.

5. *Challenges stemming from a provider's inability to recognize that normal age-related physical, social, and psychological changes in the older adult can impact the communication process are a barrier.* This barrier is being addressed via curriculum changes made to certain provider training programs that require education in human development across the life span. Some of the regulatory bodies and payor sources associated with the aging services network are beginning to require aging-related continuing education. Increasing opportunities for continuing education and self-paced learning are available via numerous learning platforms. Universities are expanding their offerings in aging-related courses and developing new certificate and gerontology degree programs. These, along with constructive changes in the way that mass media depicts older adults, should invite expanded awareness, increased cultural sensitivity, and better understanding of age-related changes.

## PREDICTIONS AND FORECASTS

The previous sections focused on aspects of the provider–older adult relationship most likely to remain unchanged and on areas where continued future improvement is forecast. While few details of the communication process itself are likely to change, what is almost certain to change are some of the topics of provider–older adult conversations, the venues where these conversations take place, and the technologies involved in the communication process. But these are not predictions, they are forecasts.

A *prediction* is a statement about what will occur. It is often authoritative and suggests certainty. A *forecast* is a statement about what might happen based on certain assumptions. It suggests probability and is conditional (Morlidge & Player, 2012). Gordon (2008) defines a "good forecast" as one that describes relevant emerging issues and discusses potential events, and that helps people prepare for specific scenarios.

A forecast could be viewed as a soft prediction—more projection than prophecy. Forecasts explore the possibility and probability of what may or may not occur based on a reasoned analysis of existing trends. This analysis is often set against a background that might include environmental, biological, and cultural variables, and is viewed through the lens of various assumptions and "what-if" scenarios. In other words, forecasts are educated guesses about some aspect of the future.

Barnatt (2012) admits the near impossibility of accurately predicting what the future may hold. He does believe that insight into possible futures can be gained by studying current challenges and trends and speculating on next-generation technologies. When it comes to predicting the future, physicist Michio Kaku (2011) insists,

> It is impossible to predict the future with complete accuracy. The best one can do, I feel, is to tap into the minds of the scientists at the cutting edge of research, who are doing the yeoman's work of inventing the future. They are the ones who are creating the devices, inventions, and therapies that will revolutionize civilization. (p. 3)

Cecily Sommers (2012) author of *Think Like a Futurist* and founder of The Push Institute (a think tank that tracks global trends) believes that significant changes in society are preceded by shifts in four major cultural forces: energy sources, advances in technology, demographic changes, and methods of governance. She refers to these interlocking forces as the four building blocks of change. The following section provides an example that illustrates Sommer's model.

1.  *The first of the four forces is new sources of energy.* Kaku (2011) envisions that by 2050, a game-changing new source of energy may become commercially available—nuclear fusion. This is thoroughly discussed in his highly recommended book *Physics of the Future: How Science will Shape Human Destiny and our Daily Lives by the year 2100.* Nuclear fusion—the process that powers the sun and stars—can provide unlimited, eternal energy from seawater. Kaku (2011) states an eight-ounce glass of seawater contains the energy equivalent to 500,000 barrels of oil. A breakthrough in harnessing nuclear fusion could provide access to levels of energy beyond anything ever before conceived, effectively ending the global "energy shortage" overnight. This new energy source would stimulate the second of the four forces—*advances in technology.*

2.  *The second force is advances in technology.* As a result of unlimited amounts of inexpensive energy generated from nuclear fusion, new technologies would be developed to deal with issues related to energy generation, storage, and transmission. The availability of unlimited energy would stimulate development of new technologies. Applications from these new technologies would ripple from industry to industry, and

converging with other technological breakthroughs, lead to the creation of more new tools, new jobs, and the creation of new wealth.

The global energy market would most likely be transformed. These changes would be temporarily disruptive to several energy-related markets—a disruption stimulating the third of the four forces—*demographics*.

3. *The third force is demographics.* The temporary disruption and rearrangement of the global energy sector and associated industries, combined with effects related to the transfer of wealth, could lead to significant changes in the makeup and location of the industries associated with energy production, storage, and distribution, and the people employed by them. These changes could have a significant impact on the world economy leading to the necessity of the fourth of the four forces—*governance*.

4. *The fourth force is governance.* To prevent, reduce, and control economic and social chaos, changes have to be managed and regulated. Governance is the major tool used to manage shifts in the first three forces, according to Sommer's model.

This example illustrates how modifications to the four forces can generate waves of change that can ripple across the surface of humanity leaving a trail of economic and social transformation in their wake.

In addition to fusion, there are many other game-changing technologies presently on the horizon and poised for penetration into the mass market. Examples include artificial intelligence, quantum computing, robotics, augmented reality, personalized genomic-based medicine, nanotechnology, and many others.

By 2100, the convergence of these technologies could lead to the creation of a society so advanced that—by present standards—it would be almost beyond recognition. Drexler (2013), in his book *Radical Abundance: How a Revolution in Nanotechnology will Change Civilization*, discusses applications of atomically precise manufacturing (APM). He predicts, "Through new technologies, human history has repeatedly changed directions, and with unimaginable consequences. The approaching APM revolution will provide the driving force for a fourth revolution, and like the preceding revolutions, it will transform daily life, labor, and the structure of society on earth" (p. 39).

All indications suggest that the society of the future will look and feel different than today's society. Using a person-centered, plain-language approach to communication, tomorrow's providers will perform a valuable service, assisting older adult clients and patients to more comfortably navigate the unknown waters of technological change.

## GOOD NEWS, BAD NEWS: EDUCATED GUESSES

First, the good news guesses: Advanced health technologies will extend the average age of populations around the globe. A new health care system is on the horizon that will help ameliorate debilitating physical and mental conditions and improve overall health and well-being (Burrows, 2012). Telehealth is on the rise. *Telehealth* is the use of "technologies to support long-distance clinical care, health education, public health and health administration" (Whitten, 2006, p. 20). As a result, greater numbers of older adults will live a healthier, longer, and more independent life than ever before in human history. The convergence of advances in fields such as nanotechnology, artificial intelligence, robotics, quantum computing, personalized medicine, and genomic-based health care, combined with cybernetic enhancement, may lead to an array of health benefits never before possible. In Japan, robots are already beginning to be used to care for select older adults (Huston, 2013).

More good news: New technologies are under development that can be used to assist older adults to successfully age in place and for increasing virtual social contact, thereby reducing isolation. Slowly changing societal attitudes combined with new economic opportunities should result in increased options for older adults—socially and economically. It is possible that new manufacturing methods based on nanotechnology and 3-D printing could usher in a twenty-first century version of a home-based industrial revolution. A new era of "working at home" could be right around the corner.

The bad news guesses: The initial impact of these changes may be socially and economically disruptive. Progress may come at considerable social and economic expense. Increased longevity may be accompanied by an increase in the number of years of dependency (Robnett & Chop, 2010). This dependency may be at least partially offset by new medical and health-related technologies.

The coming demographic shifts in population have major implications for society and especially for the aging services network. To manage the pace of change, the force of governance will have to tackle and resolve many complex challenges. Much academic, political, and public debate will ensue. Politicians and members of the public will be confronted with increasingly difficult decisions as they face questions regarding allocation of limited resources, political options, and numerous ethical conundrums. Aging services providers will also be a part of these local, state, and national debates. Effective communication will be more important than ever.

## A GLIMPSE AROUND THE BEND

When it comes to predicting technological progress, scientists have a historical record of underestimating the actual rate of progress. One classic example, provided by Kaku (2011), points out that "In 1899, Charles H. Duell, Commissioner of the US Office of Patents, said, 'Everything that can be invented has been invented'" (p. 8). Enough said.

The scientific process and accompanying accumulation of knowledge is expanding exponentially. Michio Kaku (2011)—renowned theoretical physicist and author of several best-selling books—believes it is humanity's destiny to one day live like the mythical gods of old. Metaphorically speaking, he believes the tools of computers, nanotechnology, artificial intelligence, biotechnology, and quantum theory will serve like contemporary versions of magic words, magic wands, and magic spells. Sharing his vision, he offers this interesting forecast,

> By 2100, like the gods of mythology, we will be able to manipulate objects with the power of our minds. Computers, silently reading our thoughts, will be able to carry out our wishes. We will be able to move objects by thought alone, a telekinetic power usually reserved only for the gods. With the power of biotechnology, we will create perfect bodies and extend our lifespans. We will also be able to create life forms that have never walked the surface of earth. With the power of nanotechnology, we will be able to take an object and turn it into something else, to create something seemingly almost out of nothing.
>
> *(Kaku, 2011, p. 12)*

Whatever the future may bring, it is likely that effective, person-centered provider–older adult interpersonal communication will become even more important.

The rapid aging of the global population along with its increasing economic, ethnic, and racial diversity will create new challenges and opportunities for the 59,000,000 members of the aging services network that will be impossible to predict (Stone, 2014). One thing is certain: Each person will spend the rest of his or her life in the future. This future will take place in a world that is already improving more than many realize—yet a world where significant threats remain.

## CONCLUSION

This book was born from the recognition that many older adults feel dissatisfied with the process of communicating with their providers. The purpose of this book was to introduce members of the aging services network to a person-centered, respected-based approach to communicating with older adults. It was written to share select research and data relevant to the communication process that many providers may not be aware of—information and techniques from the domains of gerontology; psychology, health psychology, and sports psychology; medicine, neuroscience, and neurocardiology; communication studies; consciousness studies; physics; and future studies.

As Glenn (2014) summarized, "The world is improving more than most pessimists know and future dangers are worse than most optimists indicate" (p. 17). Based on annual data gathered from the Millennium Project, the outlook for the future of humanity appears promising. Produced annually since 2000, the Millennium Project's forecasts are based on historical data collected on 30 key variables and the insights gathered from more than 4500 experts (Glenn, 2014). The data are clear. The overall condition of humanity is improving. Some of this improvement has been (and will likely continue to be) at a high cost to the environment. No one knows for sure how long the labor process will continue as humanity struggles to give birth to a new version of itself—humanity 2.0.

Humanity 2.0 will be a planetary civilization where about 85% of the world's population will be connected via high-speed mobile Internet by 2017. This version of humanity will be a world where advanced sensors are seamlessly and invisibly embedded in nearly every aspect of society connecting 40–80 billion "smart" devices into a planetary-wide Internet of Things by 2020 (Glenn, 2014).

As Rogers and Lalich (2014) point out, "Every five or six decades, a revolutionary technology emerges that unleashes an economic boom" (p. 13). Like it or not, an unstoppable, accelerating title wave of technological progress is about to wash over humanity. But, instead of destruction, a new world economy will most likely emerge, ushering in a new era of prosperity.

It is possible there is a new world on the horizon, a world in which the provider and the older adult could enjoy a greater awareness of the implications of the concepts of nonlocality and distance intentionality—a world inextricably interwoven and mutually influencing at the quantum level of existence combined with a technological interweaving based on an environment saturated with embedded sensors. A world of deep, underlying interconnection—a world where conscious, distance, benevolent intention is the community-based standard of care.

In the future, no matter how large a role digital virtual reality may play, the human touch will almost certainly be key in the provider–older adult relationship. As more and more online platforms and digital technologies begin to emerge, effective, respectful partnerships between providers and older adults will be needed. Providers can play a key role in helping to educate future clients and patients about how to cooperate and collaborate with providers as equal partners, in both face-to-face and virtual relationships (Mesko, 2014b).

The hope is that providers trained in person-centered, interpersonal, multicultural communication will play a significant role—now and in the future—in narrowing the intergenerational communication gap. The hope is that at a time when the entire human population will enjoy near instant access to the collective knowledge of civilization; have real-time access to artificial intelligence of genius caliber; marvel over the many creative uses of nanotechnology; and even in the face of humanoid robots, that humanity will become something more than it used to be (Glenn, 2014).

The hope is that as the Internet of People and the Internet of Things gradually intertwine and expand across the globe, humanity will feel a little more interconnected, a little more caring and compassionate—and in that moment, become more human, not less.

*Pau ka hana. Ku'ua na olelo.*

*The work is complete. Release the words.*

**Ancient Hawaiian saying**

## LIST OF MAIN POINTS FOR PREVIEW AND REVIEW

- From the first human being up through 2014, approximately 100 billion people have lived on earth. The current population is over seven billion.
- With the dawn of the Industrial Revolution and its emphasis on technological knowledge, elders lost their esteemed place in society and fell into the disempowered state that we now ascribe to a "normal" old age.
- Today, there are approximately 531 million elders—individuals aged 65 or older. This number could double by 2030 and reach over 1.5 billion by 2050.
- By 2050, the population is expected to exceed nine billion. At that time, one out of every five people will be aged 65 or older and—for the first time in history—the number of older adults will exceed those aged 15 or younger.
- Most babies born since 2000 in countries with long life expectancies such as the United States, Canada, Japan, France, Germany, Italy, and the United Kingdom will live to celebrate their one-hundredth birthday. They will be elders of the future.
- Effective communication is essential to the successful provider–older adult professional relationship. This claim was historically valid, is presently valid, and in the foreseeable future, will probably continue to be valid.

- In the future world of extreme high-tech, there will be an increased need for a respect-based, person-centered approach to interpersonal communication. Appreciation, caring, compassion, dignity, and respect are timeless virtues not likely to go out of fashion.
- While little of the communication process itself is likely to change, what is almost certain to change are some of the topics of provider–older adult conversations, the venues where these conversations take place, and the technology that is sometimes involved in the communication process.
- Improved communication can deepen rapport, increase mutual respect and understanding, enhance accurate exchange of information, improve compliance with provider recommendations, positively impact outcomes, and often save time while lowering frustration and stress for the provider and the older adult.
- The five barriers to effective, mutually satisfying communication (identified in Chapter 1) will probably continue to play a role in the provider–older adult interactions of the future.
- Predictions suggest certainty. Forecasts suggest probability. A forecast can be understood as a softer version of a prediction—more of a projection. Forecasts explore the possibility and probability of what may or may not occur based on a reasoned analysis of existing trends set against a background of environmental, biological, and cultural variables, and viewed through the lens of various "what if" scenarios.
- In the past few decades, more scientific knowledge has been discovered and accumulated than in all of human history. Within the next 75 years, scientific knowledge will have doubled from today's level, many times over.
- In the future, more individuals than ever before in human history will be living an independent, healthy, and longer life. This progress will come with considerable social and economic expense.
- More people than ever before will benefit from upcoming biomedical and technological breakthroughs. People will be confronted with increasingly difficult decisions with respect to allocation of available resources, political choices, and ethical conundrums.
- Slowly changing societal attitudes combined with new economic opportunities should result in increased opportunities for older adults for continued personal growth in later life. This increased longevity may result in an increased number of years of dependency.
- Significant challenges could arise from a population where most people live at least 100 years: the strain on personal and family finances; increased demands on the health care system, social security, and retirement funds;

ethical and political concerns surrounding allocation of limited natural resources; and challenges related to possible extended periods of dependency.

- New technological breakthroughs will continue to emerge from research into artificial intelligence, augmented reality, bioengineering, genomics, the Internet of Things, nanotechnology, personalized medicine, quantum computing, and robotics.
- When it comes to predicting technological progress, scientists routinely underestimate the rate of progress.
- Technological advances are forecasted to improve the quality of life for the twenty-first century older adult. Among other things, they could be used to enhance provider–older adult interactions, reduce social isolation, and enhance health care.
- There is a new health care system on the horizon based on personal, participatory, predictive, and preventative medicine delivered where you live. Extraordinary changes in personal monitoring devices and biotechnology are creating a world of highly individualized, preventative health care. In Japan, robots are already beginning to care for the elderly.
- Despite incredible advances, face-to-face communication challenges remain. Better technologies are being developed for "aging in place," home monitoring, communication and assessment through virtual office visits, and improved technology for increasing social contact and reducing isolation. This technology will continue to get better, faster, and cheaper.
- As online platforms and digital technologies rapidly emerge, we need partnerships between patients and health care professionals. It will become necessary to educate older adults about how to become equal partners with their providers, in both face-to-face and virtual relationships.
- There is a new world on the horizon, a world in which the provider and the older adult enjoy a greater awareness of the implications of the concepts of nonlocality and distance intentionality; a world inextricably interwoven and mutually influencing at the quantum level of existence combined with a technological interweaving based on an environment saturated with embedded sensors. This world will have a much greater level of interaction between mind and machine—a world of deep, underlying interconnection—a world where conscious, distance benevolent intention is the community-based standard of care.
- No matter how important the role that digital will play in our lives, the human touch is and will always be the key in the doctor–patient relationship.

• The world of the future will most likely be a world that embraces the reality of quantum entanglement and nonlocal distance intention—a world where deeply felt energetic and technological interconnection is the norm. This realization and experience of interconnectedness will deeply impact the individual, society, and culture. This could lead to significant changes in public education, international law and politics, and the religions of the world.

### Provider Self-Test and/or Suggestions for Instructors

**Define and discuss the key concepts:** Prediction, forecast, trends, disruptive technology, Internet of Things, nanotechnology.

**Summarize:** The changing roles of the elder from the past, to the present, and speculate on possible future roles.

**Speculate:** How communication-related technological advances might impact and improve the quality of life for the twenty-first century older adult. Include a discussion of how technology could be used to enhance provider–older adult interactions, reduce social isolation, and enhance health care.

**Discuss:** The challenges that could arise from a population where most people live at least 100 years. Discuss the potential strain on personal and family finances; increased demands on the health care system, social security, and retirement funds; ethical and political concerns surrounding allocation of limited natural resources; and challenges related to possible extended periods of dependency. Carefully examine the assumptions underlying conclusions.

**Describe:** The role of a respectful, person-centered approach in interpersonal communication in a high-tech society.

**Share:** Your vision of a world that embraces the reality of quantum entanglement and nonlocal distance intention—a world where deeply felt energetic and technological interconnection is the norm. How might this realization and experience of interconnectedness impact the individual, society, and culture? Speculate on the implications this could have on public education, international law and politics, and the religions of the world.

# WEB RESOURCES

## People

Cecily Sommers
   www.cecilysommers.com
Michio Kaku
   www.mkaku.org

## Organizations
Center for Strategic and International Studies
  http://csis.org/
Institute for Global Futures
  http://globalfuturist.com/
Institute for the Future
  http://www.iftf.org/home/
Medicalfuturist.com.
Millennium Project
  http://www.millennium-project.org/
Techcast Global
  http://www.techcastglobal.com/
United States Census
  http://www.census.gov
World Future Society
  www.wfs.org
## Journals
The Futurist: Forecasts, Trends, and Ideas about the Future.

# REFERENCES

Barnatt, C. (2012). *25 things you need to know about the future*. London, UK: Constable.
Burrows, M. (2012). *Global trends 2030: Alternative worlds*. National Intelligence Council. http://www.dni.gov/index.php/about/organization/national-intelligence-council-global-trends.
Christensen, K., Doblhammer, G., Rau, R., & Vaupel, J. W. (2009). Ageing populations: the challenges ahead. *The Lancet, 374*(9696), 1196–1208.
Drexler, K. E. (2013). *Radical abundance: How a revolution in nanotechnology will change civilization*. New York: Public Affairs.
Glenn, J. C. (2014). Our global situation and prospects for the future. *The Futurist, 48*(5), 15–20.
Gordon, A. (2008). *Future savvy: Identifying trends to make better decisions, manage uncertainty, and profit from change*. New York: AMACOM.
Huston, C. (2013). The impact of emerging technology on nursing care: Warp speed ahead. *OJIN: The Online Journal of Issues in Nursing, 18*(2).
Kaku, M. (2011). *Physics of the future: How science will shape human destiny and our daily lives by the year 2100*. New York: Anchor Books.
Mesko, B. (2014a). Rx disruption: technology trends of medicine in health care. *The Futurist, 48*(6), 7–8.
Mesko, B. (2014b). *The guide to the future of medicine: Technology and the human touch*. Elektro Press.
Morlidge, S., & Player, S. (2012). *Future ready: How to master business forecasting*. West Sussex, UK: John Wiley & Sons.
National Institute on Aging. (2011). *Talking with your older patient: A clinician's handbook*. http://www.nia.nih.gov/sites/default/files/talking_with_your_older_patient.pdf.

Robnett, R. H., & Chop, W. C. (2010). *Gerontology for the health care professional*. Subury, MA: Jones and Bartlett.

Rogers, F., & Lalich, R. (2014). *Ride the wave*. Willowbrook, IL: Crucial Trends Press.

Schachter-Shalomi, Z., & Miller, R. S. (1995). *Age-ing to sage-ing: A profound new vision of growing older*. New York: Warner Books.

Sommers, C. (2012). *Think like a futurist: Know what changes, what doesn't, and what's next*. San Francisco, CA: Jossey-Bass.

Stone, R. I. (2014). The aging services system—when it's 64. *Generations, 38*(2), 101–106.

Whitten, P. (2006). Telemedicine: communication technologies that revolutionize healthcare services. *Generations, 30*(2), 20–24.

World Health Organization. (2011). *Global Health and Aging*. http://www.who.int/ageing/publications/global_health.pdf.

# INDEX

*Note:* Page numbers with "b" indicate boxes.

Edwards Brothers Malloy
Thorofare, NJ  USA
June 11, 2015